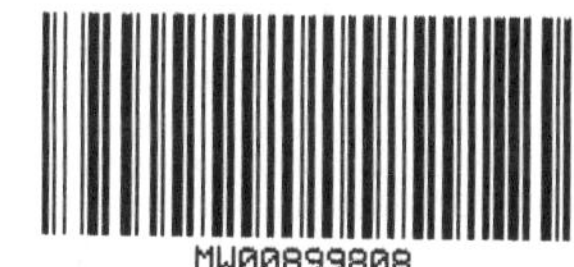

NO-STRESS ANTI-INFLAMMATORY COOKBOOK

for Beginners

Tasty Recipes with Powerful Natural Ingredients to Boost Immunity, Reduce Inflammation & Detox Your Body.16-Week Meal Plan

Full Meals in Just 20 minutes!

By

Alison Tenny

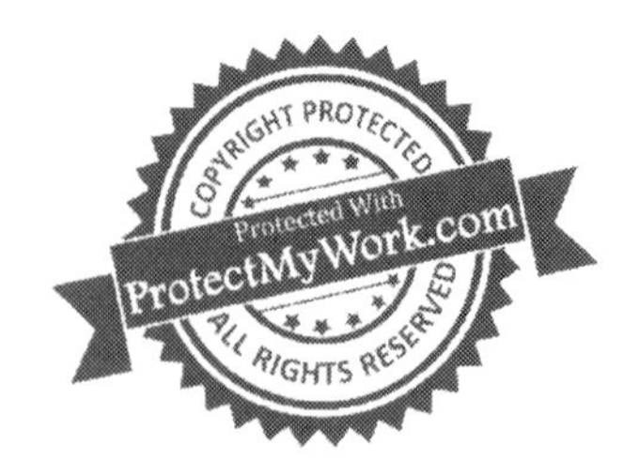
COPYRIGHT PROTECTED
Protected With
ProtectMyWork.com
ALL RIGHTS RESERVED

❋ YOUR EXCLUSIVE BONUSES AWAITS! ❋

Thank you for investing in your health with our book! As a token of our appreciation, we're gifting you an additional GUIDE and a very useful SHOPPING CARD!

❋ **BONUS 1:**

"FLAME-OFF: Your 5-Step NO-STRESS Anti-Inflammatory Blueprint"

EVERYTHING YOU NEED BEYOND THE RECIPE BOOK!

Have you ever wondered about the natural secrets that could help you live a healthier, inflammation-free life? Inside this book, we've crafted an exclusive bonus just for you. A compelling guide that unveils the essential steps to an anti-inflammatory lifestyle.

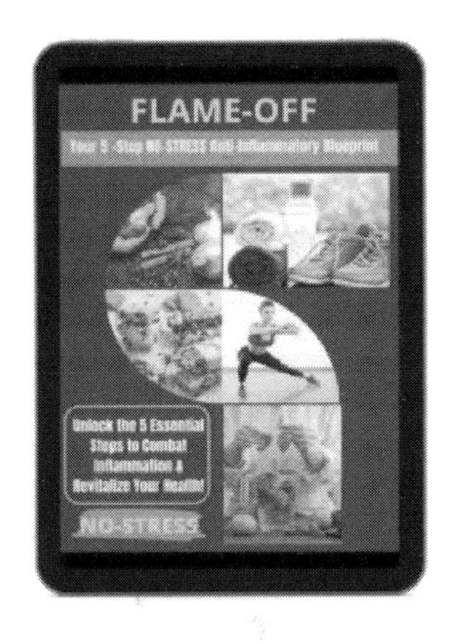

Here's what awaits:

Tried-and-True Strategies: Dive into techniques that have aided thousands in finding relief and wellness.

Key Skills: Unearth the pivotal competencies that can reshape your health and well-being.

Journey of Discovery: Brace yourself to explore and embrace new habits that can turn your health around.

❋ **BONUS 2:**

A Very Useful Shopping Card Is Waiting for You!

Don't let this exclusive content slip away.

Head To the Designated Bonus Section NOW and Claim Your Comprehensive Guide and a Shopping Card.

<u>You've earned it!</u>

TABLE OF CONTENTS

Introduction

When something foreign enters your body like a germ, plant pollen or a chemical your immune system kick, into gear. This often leads to inflammation. Inflammation serves as a response to fight off invaders and keep you healthy. However, there are times when inflammation occurs without any foreign substances present. In cases inflammation can actually work against you. Free radicals are a class of molecules that can cause damage to cells and increase the risk of inflammatory disorders.

Enough the effective way to combat inflammation is through food rather than medication. Chemicals in some meals can cause or aggravate inflammation. Opting for nutritious meals over processed or sugary foods reduces the likelihood of contributing to inflammation. Including plenty of fruits and vegetables in your diet is crucial for a inflammatory approach as they are rich in antioxidants that help neutralize harmful substances in the body.

However it's worth noting that some foods have the potential to generate radicals when cooked in oil. Free radicals harm cells and exacerbate inflammation-related diseases.

To counteract these radicals and their damaging effects on your bodys cells antioxidants play a role by eliminating them. Our daily activities like metabolism naturally produce radicals within our bodies. Additionally factors such, as stress and smoking can further increase their presence. By reducing activity through antioxidants action we minimize cell damage and subsequently reduce the chances of experiencing inflammation related health problems.

However it's important to note that consuming antioxidants can be beneficial because they assist the body in getting rid of toxins. When following a diet aimed at reducing inflammation it's best to prioritize foods that have inflammatory properties, over those that generate free radicals. For instance, oily salmon's omega-3 fatty acids can help cut protein intake.

To make your transition to a diet easier here are some suggestions; Start by incorporating a variety of fruits, vegetables and wholesome snacks into your shopping list. Gradually replace food with home cooked meals over time. Consider swapping drinks for mineral water or other healthier alternatives. Before taking any supplements like cod liver oil or multivitamins it's always an idea to consult with your doctor first. Every day, you should aim to do some light physical activity for at least 30 minutes. Remember that maintaining sleep hygiene is crucial since lack of sleep can actually worsen inflammation. If you're dealing with conditions that could be aggravated by inflammation following an anti-inflammatory diet, as a complementary treatment might be beneficial.

Chapter 1: Anti-Inflammatory Diet

The anti-inflammatory diet has gained significant popularity in recent times. It's more than just a fleeting trend. To foster a balanced inflammatory response in our bodies, the primary step in embracing this diet is to prioritize whole, natural, and unprocessed foods. By doing so, we can effectively reduce inflammation, thereby decreasing the risks of conditions such as fibromyalgia, heart disease, cancer, chronic pain, and persistent dyspepsia.

Let's dive deeper into understanding inflammation and the reasons we aim to manage it. Consider the last time you became ill or hurt yourself physically. These incidents, which undeniably involve inflammation, are the body's responses to external challenges like injuries or illnesses. Normally, this reaction diminishes once the root cause is resolved. Yet, if inflammation lingers far beyond its initial trigger, it can become problematic.

To encourage a healthy inflammatory response, it's beneficial to regularly incorporate vibrant fruits, vegetables, herbs, spices, and healthy fats into our diets. On the flip side, limiting or avoiding potential inflammatory triggers is equally important. Foods such as refined carbohydrates (like crackers, cakes, and bagels), gluten-laden products, sugary dishes, and those fried in trans fats are recognized contributors to inflammation.

1.1 What is the definition of inflammation?

The inflammatory response is perfectly normal and necessary for the body's recovery. It's essentially how the body delivers nutrients and boosts immune activity to infected or injured areas.

The immune system triggers an inflammatory reaction in response to exposure to a pathogen or tissue injury. For instance, if you cut your finger, inflammation might cause it to become red and swollen. This is helpful because it promotes more circulation to repair broken tissues. Pain is the body's way of telling us when something is wrong. Prostaglandins, prostacyclins, thromboxanes, and leukotrienes are all eicosanoids, and they're all involved in fighting off infections and healing wounds. Normally, after the threat is addressed, anti-inflammatory compounds are produced to regulate the immune response.

Chronic inflammation can manifest as a variety of symptoms, including:

- Body aches and pains
- Persistent stiffness
- Loss of joint function
- Consistent swelling
- Ongoing indigestion
- Regular diarrhea
- Frequent blemishes on the skin

Over time, chronic inflammation is like a slow poison, doing havoc on your body by way of hyperactive inflammatory molecules.

In addition to the aforementioned, other diseases associated with persistent inflammation include:

- Allergies
- Asthma
- Cancer
- Crohn's disease, a chronic inflammatory bowel disorder
- Fibromyalgia
- Irritable bowel syndrome (IBD)
- Heart issues
- Kidney disease
- Psoriasis
- Rheumatoid arthritis (RA)

Inflammation-Producing Foods

Research indicates that diet is a primary contributor to chronic inflammation. Some foods can incite inflammation in the body, and regular consumption of these can lead to chronic inflammation. Avoiding inflammatory meals is just as crucial as eating items that reduce inflammation.

Advanced Glycation End-Products (AGEs)

AGEs, or advanced glycation end products, are inflammatory byproducts of normal metabolic processes. AGEs are formed during food preparation and are not naturally occurring. It's believed that all AGEs induce inflammation, irrespective of their origin.

- AGEs are abundant in heavily processed foods like frankfurters, bacon, and egg white powder.
- Examples of preserved and pasteurized prepackaged items include white flour, cake mixes, processed cereals, dry milk, dried eggs, pasteurized milk, canned or frozen pre-cooked meals, mayonnaise, cream cheese, butter, margarine, and pasteurized dried fruits.

Trans Fatty Acids

- Tran's fats are the most inflammatory of all fats.
- Inflammatory prostaglandins are produced in response to these lipids.
- Fried and deep-fried dishes, typically cooked in hydrogenated shortening, contain trans fats. Margarine and shortening also contain high levels of trans fats.
- Dairy-free creamers
- Biscuits
- Baked items like cakes, pie crusts, and cookies (especially those with icing)
- Snack items like crackers and chips that list hydrogenated oils as an ingredient.

1.2 Foods That Cause Inflammation

Omega-6 fatty acids, certain meats, full-fat dairy, and eggs can be a double-edged sword. On one side, they're packed with vital vitamins and minerals; on the other, they come with saturated fats that might crank up our inflammatory markers. There's evidence, for example, that these fats can spike fibrinogen and CRP levels in our blood, hinting at increased inflammation.

Omega-6 Fatty Acids: They're a bit tricky. While they're unsaturated and essential in the right amounts, going overboard can open a Pandora's box of health issues. Think inflammation, problematic blood clotting, and even potential unchecked cell growth. The root of the problem? Our diets often lean heavily on meats and vegetable oils like corn, safflower, soybean, and cottonseed - all chock full of omega-6. And guess where these oils often lurk? Processed and fast foods.

Nightshades: They're nutritional powerhouses but come with a tiny asterisk. Some folks might find that these veggies and fruits - we're talking potatoes, tomatoes, eggplants, ground cherries, and tomatillos - can ramp up inflammation. It's all about how they interact with individual body.

1.3 Inflammation-Reducing Foods

Fortunately, there are foods that can help combat inflammation in your body. Interestingly some of the remedies for reducing inflammation can be found not in pharmacies but in grocery stores. To discover food options, it's advisable to explore the outer edges of the supermarket. It’s recommended to incorporate a variety of colored produce herbs, spices and foods rich in healthy fats into your diet. Let's talk about the anti-inflammatory essentials you can't live without.

Fruits and vegetables play a role in combating inflammation as they contain phytochemicals and antioxidants. Plants include substances called phytochemicals that provide health advantages such lowering the risk of diabetes, heart disease, and cancer. These compounds are vital for plants defense mechanisms against radicals, prolonged sun exposure, as well as bacterial and fungal infections. When we consume these plant compounds through our diet they provide protection by permeating our body tissues.

Omega 3 fatty acids have been shown to reduce inflammation. These fatty acids give rise to eicosanoids. Molecules, with hormone properties. The two most important omega 3 eicosanoids are eicosapentaenoic acid (EPA) and docosahexaenoic acid (DHA). The advantages of EPA and DHA include widening blood vessels preventing blood clotting and reducing inflammation. Omega 3s can be found in fish with a lot of fat, like salmon, striped sea bass, wild albacore tuna, and sardines.

Probiotics

Omega 3s can also be found in walnuts, soybeans, tofu and flaxseed. The human body naturally hosts a range of beneficial bacteria. Although bacteria often have a reputation certain strain like lactobacilli and Bifidobacterium actually contribute to maintaining good health and defending against diseases. These microbes help strengthen the system to fight off infections effectively.Constipation, diarrhoea, inflammatory bowel disease (IBD), and irritable bowel syndrome (IBS) are all illnesses that can be helped by their anti-inflammatory effects in the intestines. By consuming foods that're rich in beneficial probiotics like Lactobacillus acidophilus you can promote the growth of healthy bacteria in your digestive tract. Fermented dairy products like yogurt, kefir and certain soy based beverages can increase the number of probiotic bacteria in both your gut and throughout your body. Make sure to choose products labeled as "live and active cultures" for maximum intake of these bacteria.

Light Protein Options

Options When it comes to lean protein sources opt for meats such as poultry, without skin and eggs since they contain lower levels of fats that cause inflammation. Cold water fish not provide protein but also offer anti-inflammatory omega 3 fatty acids.

Vegetable proteins, such as soy products, beans, lentils, whole grains, seeds and nuts have the ability to reduce inflammatory agents in the body. In addition to this, they supply a wide variety of phytochemicals and antioxidants, both of which are good for our health.

Garlic

The inflammatory properties of garlic are well known. It contains compounds that help alleviate inflammation in the body. Because of this, eating garlic may help alleviate the discomfort and inflammation caused by illnesses such as asthma, rheumatoid arthritis, and osteoarthritis.

Curcumin

Curcumin Turmeric gets its distinctive yellow hue from curcumin. Curcumin has potential anti-inflammatory, anti-cancer, and antioxidant effects. Initial studies conducted on animals show results regarding curcumins anti-inflammatory and anticancer effects. But further study is needed to see if it might help humans avoid sickness.

Ginger

Ginger is a spice closely related to turmeric. One of its components called gingerols has shown potential in suppressing the production of substances in the body. Because of this, ginger can be used for the treatment of inflammatory disorders including rheumatoid arthritis and osteoarthritis You can add ginger to stir fries or dipping sauces to enhance your meals with a tangy and slightly sweet flavor.

1.4 Anti-Inflammatory Diet's Advantages

Research has indicated that following a diet that reduces inflammation can be beneficial in managing illness symptoms. Atherosclerosis, which is when plaque builds up in the arteries, is one of the most common of these. Individuals with type 2 diabetes may find relief from inflammatory markers by adhering to an anti-inflammatory diet as studies have uncovered a connection between subclinical atherosclerosis and cardiovascular disease mortality. Those who strictly follow the Mediterranean diet, which shares similarities with the anti-inflammatory diet, tend to experience fewer symptoms related to inflammation compared to those who don't.

The Mediterranean diet emphasizes protein meals and low-fat dairy products while favoring plant-based proteins like beans, nuts, and seeds. Including a variety of fruits and vegetables in our diets is important as they provide essential antioxidants that help combat inflammation and maintain consistent energy levels. An anti-inflammatory diet should also include vitamins and minerals, healthy fats, fiber, and phytonutrients.

By adopting an anti-inflammatory diet approach, individuals may potentially prevent excessive weight gain since this dietary approach discourages excessive calorie consumption that can lead to fat accumulation and obesity. There may be connections between consuming a pro-inflammatory diet and obesity. One diet that can cause inflammation includes eating refined carbohydrates, processed meats, and junk food.

These foods are low in calories and fiber which means people may need to eat more of them to make up for the lack of fullness. Furthermore, people following this diet tend to be less active which leads to consuming more calories and being less physically active. People who are already sick often benefit the most from an anti-inflammatory diet. Such diets avoid sugars and carbohydrates as they are linked to conditions like type 2 diabetes, metabolic syndrome, and obesity. For example, an anti-inflammatory diet promotes the consumption of rice because it is high in fiber and has a low glycemic index.

Over time, the health benefits of adopting an anti-inflammatory diet become apparent. It's important to eat less saturated and trans fats and more omega-3 fatty acids. Heart diseases are more likely to happen when you eat a lot of fat. The accumulation of lipids on blood vessel linings can lead to narrowing arteries and high blood pressure. This can result in damage to blood vessels and other organs when the heart has to work to pump blood. Heart-healthy oils, like olive oil and flaxseed oil, are recommended in an anti-inflammatory diet.

Therefore, it is crucial to maintain a diet that's low in inflammatory foods to ensure healthy blood pressure in the long run. In addition, a diet aimed at reducing inflammation can also help address feelings of fatigue. When our immune system becomes overly active, it can lead to increased levels of histamine resulting in drowsiness, fatigue, and irritability. Fatigue is the body's way of signaling the need for rest and recovery due to the system's actions. However, following an anti-inflammatory diet can help alleviate or even eliminate this fatigue. Even though it's not directly linked to fat, a diet that fights inflammation can help you lose weight.

Even if someone is not classified as obese, they may still be overweight or on their way towards obesity. The increase in consumption of carbohydrates and sugars has been attributed to unintended weight gain along with other factors like a sedentary lifestyle. Diets high in carbohydrates lack essential nutrients and often lead to higher calorie intake in order to meet energy requirements.

Furthermore, the lack of fiber in diets can leave people feeling unsatisfied even after consuming large amounts of food. Fortunately, an anti-inflammatory diet promotes nutrient-rich foods while minimizing refined carbs, thus avoiding potentially harmful sugars and carbohydrates.

Making choices that reduce inflammation offers various indirect benefits as well. Reducing inflammation can have an impact on overall well-being as it often leads to discomfort, tiredness, swelling, and limited mobility. These symptoms can disrupt our routines, causing us to miss work or school. Making changes aimed at reducing inflammation can help us focus better on our educational or professional goals.

Another advantage of consuming anti-inflammatory foods is improved sleep. Our diet can affect the quality and patterns of our sleep. The consumption of foods that promote inflammation can lead to reduced sleep quality as well as disrupted sleep patterns.

Issues like excessive snacking can negatively affect both the duration and quality of our sleep. Feeling exhausted may sometimes require taking naps. However, adopting an anti-inflammatory diet that ensures a balanced intake of calories and nutrients can promote better sleep.

Lastly, an anti-inflammatory diet encourages diversity and choice in food selection, making it a versatile option for different dietary plans. This type of diet provides vitamins, minerals, and calories that help reduce or eliminate inflammation. It shares similarities with diets like veganism and the Mediterranean diet.

Having flexibility in decision-making is crucial for the success of any plan, and the anti-inflammatory diet offers just that by considering factors such as cost, cultural preferences, and seasonal availability when making choices.

1.5 Complementary Concepts - Alkalinity and Glycemic Index

Within the vast realm of nutrition, the anti-inflammatory diet stands out as a beacon for health. As we journey deeper, it's worth noting some parallel concepts that might complement our primary approach: the idea of dietary alkalinity and the significance of the glycemic index. Without diverging from our main focus, let's quickly touch upon these concepts.

Alkalinity and Inflammation

Certain substances, according to the alkaline diet, can alter the pH equilibrium of our bodies. While our body tightly regulates its pH, proponents believe that leaning towards alkaline foods can support overall health and possibly complement the effects of an anti-inflammatory diet. Foods like green leafy vegetables, almonds, and beetroot are often highlighted in this approach. Remember, the idea isn't to shift entirely but to be aware and possibly integrate some of these foods.

Glycemic Index: A Glimpse

The glycemic index (GI) measures how swiftly foods raise our blood sugar. Foods with a high GI can cause abrupt increases in blood sugar, which may aggravate inflammation. On the other hand, low-GI foods, like whole grains, nuts, and legumes, offer sustained energy and may support our anti-inflammatory endeavors. It's beneficial to recognize high versus low GI foods and make informed choices that align with our health goals.

Marrying the Concepts

While the anti-inflammatory diet remains paramount, understanding alkalinity and glycemic index offers supplementary tools for a well-rounded approach. They're not the centerpiece, but side notes to enrich our nutritional repertoire. As we navigate the world of anti-inflammatory foods, sprinkling in some knowledge from these ideas can beneficial.

Concluding and Next with the Recipes

Here we are at the end of this informative journey on anti-inflammatory nutrition. Through the preceding pages, we've delved together into the intricacies of inflammation, learning not just its causes, but also the ways we can counteract it through mindful food choices.

We've outlined the importance and pivotal role of inflammation in our body. As we've seen, it's a defense mechanism, but if not kept in check, can turn into a silent foe causing various ailments.

We also touched on foods: those to avoid, which are responsible for triggering or exacerbating inflammation, and those to prioritize, helping our body maintain health and balance. And, albeit briefly, we touched upon the concept of alkalinity and the glycemic index, giving you a taste of the many facets, the world of nutrition has to offer.

Now, theory is undeniably essential, but as the saying goes, "practice makes perfect." And what better way to put into practice what we've learned than through delicious recipes?

This brings us to the heart of our cookbook, a collection of dishes designed to seamlessly integrate the concept of an anti-inflammatory diet into daily life. It's not just about eating to be well, but also about savoring, celebrating, and experimenting in the kitchen. Each recipe was crafted with not just health in mind, but also taste, demonstrating that "healthy" and "tasty" can indeed go hand in hand.

So, are you ready to don your apron and hit the stove? The recipes will guide you step by step, introducing you to perhaps new ingredients and combinations, but always with flavor and well-being in mind.

Good luck and... ENJOY YOUR MEAL!

Chapter 2: Breakfast Recipes

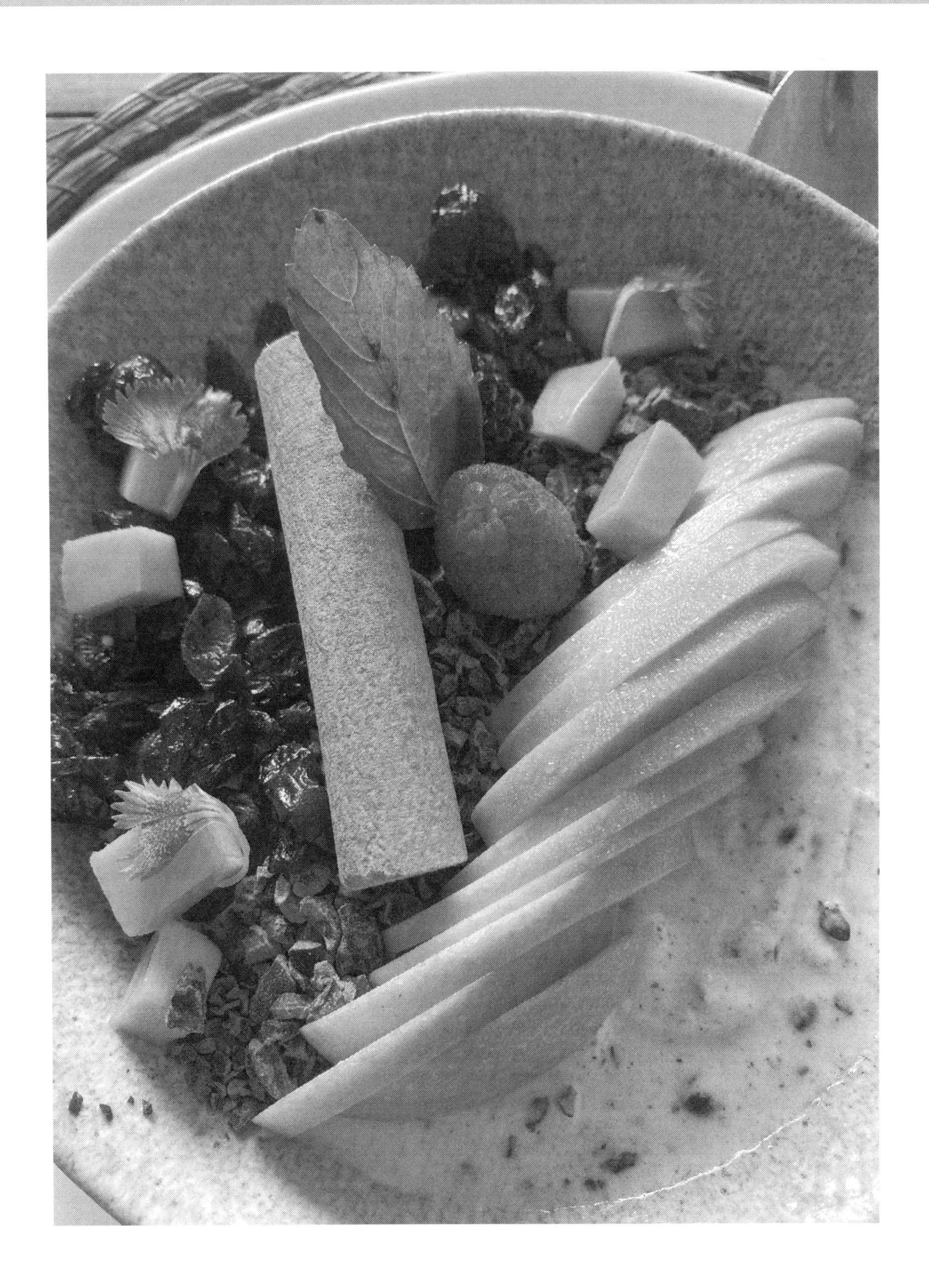

2.1. Egg Kale with Casserole

Ready In:

- Prep: 8 Min
- Cook: 25 Min
- Yields: 6

What you need:

- 1 tbsp avocado oil
- 5 fresh kale leaves, torn into pieces
- 1 garlic clove, (minced)
- ½ tsp salt, divided
- 1 onion, chopped
- 9 large eggs (beaten)
- 2 tbsp lemon juice
- 1½ tsp rosemary
- 1 tsp oregano
- ¼ tsp ground black(pepper)
- 2 tbsp water
- ½ cup nutritional yeast

Directions:

1. In a big pan over medium heat, warm the avocado oil. Once hot, add the onions and sauté for about 2 to 3 minutes.
2. Add cabbage, lemon juice, garlic, and pinch of salt. Stir until cabbage begins to wilt, about 2/3 minutes.
3. Eggs, water, the remaining salt, pepper, rosemary, oregano, and nutritional yeast are whisked together in a mixing dish.
4. Fold the sautéed kale and onions into the egg mixture.
5. Transfer to a pre-greased casserole dish.
6. Set oven temperature to 375°F.
7. Bake the casserole for 20-25 minutes, or until firm and golden on top.
8. Allow to cool and serve.

Nutritional Info:

Calories: 47 | Carbs: 7g | Protein: 1,3g | Fat: 1.2g | Sodium: 21mg

2.2. Raspberry Steel Cut Oatmeal Bars

Ready In:

- Prep: 5 Min
- Cook: 40 Min
- Yields: 6.

What you need:

- 3 cups steel-cut oats
- 3 eggs
- 2 cups vanilla almond milk
- 1 cup frozen raspberries
- ⅓ cup erythritol
- ¼ tsp salt
- 1 tsp vanilla extract
- Cooking spray or oil for the pan
-

Directions:

1. Turn on the oven and bring it to 375°F.
2. In a pot, heat vanilla almond milk until simmering. Cook oats for about 20 minutes (should be soft)
3. In another bowl, combine eggs, erythritol, vanilla, and salt.
4. Mix the oat mixture with the egg mixture, then add raspberries.
5. Grease a baking dish, pour in the oat mixture, spreading evenly.
6. Set in the oven for around 20 minutes.
7. Wait until it has cooled down before slicing it up and serving it.

Nutritional Info:

Calories: 48 | Carbs: 5g | Protein: 4g | Fat: 1.1g | Sodium: 23mg

2.3. Blueberry Vanilla Quinoa Porridge

Ready In:

- Prep: 1 Min
- Cook: 15 Min
- Yields: 6

What you need:

- 1½ cups dry quinoa
- 3 cups water
- 1 cup frozen blueberries
- ½ tsp stevia powder
- 1 tsp vanilla extract

Directions:

1. Rinse the quinoa thoroughly until the water runs clear.
2. Bring water to a boil in a pot, add the quinoa, reduce the heat, cover, and simmer for 10-12 minutes.
3. Add blueberries, stevia, and vanilla, and cook for a few more minutes until everything is soft.
4. Allow to cool and serve.

Nutritional Facts:

Calories: 47 | Carbs: 8g | Protein: 1.2g | Fat: 1.3g | Sodium: 21mg

2.4. Buckwheat Ginger Granola

Ready In:

- Prep: 8 Min
- Cook: 25 Min
- Yields: 8

What you need:

- 1½ cups buckwheat groats
- ⅓ cup shredded coconut
- ⅓ cup walnuts (chopped)
- ¼ cup liquid coconut oil
- 1½ cups rolled oats
- A thumb of ginger, finely grated
- 3 tbsp date syrup
- 1 tsp cinnamon
- a pinch of salt

Directions:

1. Preheat your oven to 350°F (175°C).
2. In a large bowl, combine buckwheat, oats, walnuts, and coconut.
3. Drizzle in coconut oil, ginger, date syrup, cinnamon, and salt, ensuring everything is well-coated.
4. After lining a baking sheet with baking paper, spread the ingredients in an even layer.
5. Bake for 20-25 minutes, stirring the pan occasionally to ensure even baking.
6. When finished baking, take it out of the oven and let it cool down.

Info. Nutritional:

Calories: 44 | Carbs: 4g | Protein: 5 g | Fat: 2g | Sodium: 27mg

2.5. Triple Berry Steel Cut Oats

Ready In:

- Prep: 5 Min.
- Cook: 25-30 Min.
- Yields: 6 Hearty Servings

What you need:

- 2 cups steel-cut oats
- 3 cups unsweetened almond milk
- 3 cups water
- 1 tsp vanilla extract
- ⅓ cup monk fruit sweetener
- ¼ tsp salt
- 1½ cups frozen berry medley (strawberries, blackberries, raspberries)

Directions:

1. In a pot, mix almond milk and water, and bring to a gentle boil.
2. Reduce heat and simmer for 20 minutes, stirring occasionally.
3. Stir in vanilla, monk fruit sweetener, salt, and frozen berries.
4. Continue heating for 5-10 minutes until oats are creamy.
5. Serve with almond milk, almonds, or fresh berries, if desired.

Nutritional Info: Calories: 224 | Carbs: 42g | Protein: 7g | Fat: 3g | Sodium: 130mg

2.6. Banana Pancake Muffins

Ready In:

- Prep: 8 Min.
- Cook: 15-18 Min.
- Yields:3

What you need:

- 3 ripe bananas
- 3 eggs
- 2 tbsp erythritol
- 1¾ cups rolled oats
- Pinch of cinnamon
- Dash of vanilla essence
- 1 tsp baking powder

Directions:

1. Turn on and bring the oven to 350°F (175°C).
2. Blend oats, bananas, eggs, cinnamon, vanilla, erythritol, and baking powder until smooth.
3. Fill muffin tin or silicone cups three-quarters full.
4. Bake until golden, check with a toothpick for doneness.
5. Cool briefly before removing.

Nutritional Facts: Calories: 204 | Carbs: 33g | Protein: 5g | Fat: 8g | Sodium: 120mg

2.7. Cinnamon-Flax Morning Bread

Ready In:

- Prep: 6 Min
- Cook: 35-40 Min.
- Serve For: 6

What you need:

- ½ cup almond flour
- ½ cup flaxseed meal
- Generous sprinkle of cinnamon
- Pinch of salt
- ⅔ cup xylitol
- 2 tsp baking powder
- 4 eggs
- ½ cup melted coconut oil

Directions:

1. Turn on oven to 350F (175C).
2. Combine xylitol, baking soda, salt, and cinnamon with almond flour, flaxseed, and baking powder in a bowl.
3. In a different bowl, beat the eggs with the melted coconut oil.
4. Add to the dry stuff and mix.
5. Bake until fragrant.
6. Let cool, then slice and serve.

Nutritional Facts: Calories: 324 | Carbs: 10g | Protein: 6g | Fat: 29g | Sodium: 120mg

2.8. Veggie Morning Delight

Ready In:

- Prep: 8 Min.
- Cook: 25 Min
- Serve For: 2

What you need:

- 2 tbsp avocado oil
- 3 thinly sliced leeks (light green and white sections only)
- 8 oz mushrooms, sliced
- Pinch of salt and pepper
- 2 carrots, sliced
- 5 kale leaves, (chopped)
- Juice from half a lemon

Directions:

1. Heat avocado oil in a skillet over medium heat.
2. Add leeks, mushrooms, salt, and pepper. Sauté for 10 minutes.
3. Add carrots and cook for 5 more minutes.
4. Stir in kale and lemon juice.
5. Serve hot, optionally with seeds or a soft-boiled egg.

Nutritional Facts: Calories: 200 | Carbs: 27g | Protein: 17g | Fat: 8g | Sodium: 150mg

2.9. Rustic Root Veggie & Egg Bake

Ready In:

- Prep: 15 Min.
- Cook: 30-35 Min.
- Serve For: 4

What you need:

- 1 onion, diced
- 1 turnip, diced
- 1 parsnip, diced
- 2 carrots, diced
- 1 tbsp avocado oil
- 1 tsp kosher salt
- 1 onion, diced
- 8 eggs, whisked
- 1 tbsp lemon juice
- Handful of fresh thyme leaves

Directions:

1. Preheat oven to 375°F (190°C).
2. Sauté onion, turnip, parsnip, carrots, and salt in heated avocado oil until tender.
3. Mix eggs, lemon juice, cooked veggies, and thyme in a bowl.
4. Pour into an ovenproof dish and bake until set.
5. Let it cool slightly, then slice and serve.

Nutritional Facts: Calories: 204 | Carbs: 15g | Protein: 8g | Fat: 6g | Sodium: 175mg

2.10. Creamy Strawberry Quinoa Delight

Ready In:

- Prep: 5 Min.
- Cook: 15-20 Min.
- Yields: 6

What you need:

- 1 can (13.66-oz) full-fat coconut milk
- 1½ cups quinoa (rinse before use)
- 1½ cups water
- 1½ cups quinoa (rinse before use)
- ½ tsp stevia powder
- 1 tsp vanilla extract
- ⅓ cup unsweetened coconut shreds
- 1 cup strawberry slices

Directions:

1. Rinse quinoa thoroughly.
2. In a pot, combine quinoa, water, coconut milk, stevia, and vanilla. Heat until bubbling, then reduce to simmer for 15-20 minutes.
3. Fold in strawberries.
4. Cool slightly, serve, and sprinkle with coconut shreds.

Nutritional Facts: Calories: 174 | Carbs: 22g | Protein: 6g | Fat: 8g | Sodium: 125mg

2.11. Quick Egg & Asparagus Breakfast

Ready In:

- Prep: 8 Min.
- Cook: 20 Min.
- Yields: 6

What you need:

- 1 can (13.66-oz) lush full-fat coconut milk
- 1½ cups quinoa (always rinse before using)
- 1½ cups water
- ½ tsp stevia powder for a touch of sweetness
- 1 tsp aromatic vanilla extract
- 1 cup juicy strawberry slices
- ⅓ cup coconut shreds (unsweetened)

Steps:

1. Begin with a quinoa rinse to ditch any bitterness.
2. In a pot, mix quinoa, water, coconut milk, stevia, and vanilla until they're all friends.
3. Heat until bubbly, then simmer and cover for 15-20 minutes until quinoa is ready and the liquid's gone.
4. Fold in the strawberries.
5. Let it cool for a moment, serve, and dust with coconut shreds.

Nutritional Facts:

Calories: 180 | carbohydrates: 23 g | Protein: 7 g | Fat: 8 g | Sodium: 125 mg

2.11. Quick Egg & Asparagus Breakfast

Ready In:

- Prep Time: 2 Min.
- Cook Time: 12 Min.
- Yields: 1 (Abundant)

What you need:

- 2 eggs
- 5 asparagus spears (break off those tough bits)

Steps:

1. Bring water to a boil, enough to cozy up to the eggs.
2. Use a spoon for the egg introduction. Boil for about 10 minutes or adjust for preferred yolk consistency.
3. Simultaneously, steam the asparagus for 3-5 minutes, leaving a hint of crunch.
4. Have an icy bath ready for the eggs. Post-boil, let them chill, then peel.
5. Plate up with the eggs cozying up to the asparagus.

Nutritional Facts:

Calories: 124 | Carbs: 6 g | Protein: 17 g | Fat: 9 g | Sodium: 100 mg

2.12. Morning Bliss: Fruit & Seed Bars

Ready In:

- Prep: 5 Min.
- Bake: 20 Min. |
- Yields: 12 Squares (6 Servings)

What you need:

- ½ cup date pieces (no pits)
- ¾ cup sunflower seeds (nicely roasted)
- ¾ cup pumpkin seeds (also roasted)
- ¾ cup white sesame seeds
- ½ cup dried blueberries
- ½ cup dried cherries
- ¼ cup flaxseed
- ½ cup almond butter (that nutty goodness)

Steps:

1. Get your oven to 325°F. Prepare an 8x8-inch baking dish with some parchment paper.
2. Utilizing a food processor, make a paste out of the dates.
3. Throw in the seeds and fruits, pulse to combine.
4. Mix this with the almond butter in another bowl.
5. Press this mix into your baking dish and bake until it has a golden hue - roughly 20 minutes.
6. Let it chill, then carve into 12 tempting squares.

Nutritional Facts:

Calories: 144 | Carbs: 28 g | Protein: 7 g | Fat: 15 g | Sodium: 120 mg

2.13. Wake-Up Call: Coconut-Chia Pudding

Ready In:

- Prep: 5 Min
- Chill Time: 30 Minutes Or Dream The Night Away |
- Yields: 4 Refreshing Servings

What you need:

- ¾ cup water (refreshing)
- ¾ cup unsweetened almond milk (silky smooth)
- 1 tsp vanilla essence (a drop of magic)
- ¼ cup chia seeds (the tiny powerhouses)
- ¼ cup coconut shreds (sun-kissed and unsweetened)
- 2 tbsp honey (nature's sweet hug)
- ½ cup strawberries (sliced to perfection)

Steps:

1. Grab a bowl and swirl in water, almond milk, and your dash of vanilla magic.
2. Let chia seeds dive in and stir the ensemble. Park it in the fridge - a short half-hour for the impatient or all night for a tomorrow treat.
3. Once your mix has transformed, swirl in coconut and honey for that morning kiss.
4. Serve in bowls and jazz up with strawberry slices. Delish!

Nutritional Facts:

Calories: 124 | Carbs: 14 g | Protein: 8 g | Fat: 8 g | Sodium: 120 mg

2.14. Sunny Morning Coconut Pancakes

Ready In:
Prep: 6 Min.
Cook: 10 Min.
Yields: 4

What you need:

- 1 tsp baking powder (fluff factor)
- 4 eggs (nature's binders)
- ½ cup almond flour (the nutty base)
- ⅓ cup unsweetened almond milk (silky)
- 2 tbsp honey (because mornings need love)
- ¼ cup coconut flour (tropical vibes)
- 1 tsp vanilla extract (another hint of magic)
- Coconut oil for frying (keep it tropical)

Steps:

1. Whisk the flours and baking powder in a bowl.
2. Welcome the eggs, almond milk, honey, and vanilla to the party. Stir until just combined.
3. Fire up the stove to medium heat. Coconut oil graces your pan for each pancake batch.
4. Pour small circles and cook till bubbles pop up and then flip.
5. Stack them high and serve. Drizzle some extra honey or top with your fave fruits.

Nutritional Facts:

Calories: 200 | Carbs: 15 g | Protein: 9 g | Fat: 13 g | Sodium: 100 mg

2.15. Rise & Shine Rice Porridge

Ready In:
Prep: 10 Min.
Cook: 20–25 Min.
Yields Two Abundant

What You'll Need:

- A pair of sweet dates, chopped up
- 1 oz. of your favorite unflavored protein powder
- A generous 1 ½ cups of almond milk
- ½ cup of those cozy short grain brown rice grains
- 1 banana, cut into lovely slices
- A spoonful of creamy tahini
- An apple, cut into bite-sized pieces
- A sprinkle of toasted sesame seeds

Steps:

1. Grab a pot and mix the rice, almond milk, and protein powder.
2. Set your stove to medium heat and cook for 20–25 minutes, stirring occasionally.
3. Add in the dates, banana slices, and apple chunks and stir.
4. Plate your porridge, drizzle with tahini and sprinkle with sesame seeds.

Nutritional Facts

Calories: 140 | Carbs: 30g | Protein: 8 g | Fat: 1.9 g | Sodium: 120 mg

2.16. Maple-Cinnamon Quinoa Delight

Ready In:
Prep: 5 Min.
Cook:15 Min.
Serve For: 4

What You'll Need:

- Non-dairy milk, 1 cup, unsweetened
- 1 cup well-rinsed quinoa
- 1 tsp of cinnamon
- 1 cup water
- ¼ cup of crunchy pecans (or your choice of nut/seed)
- 2 tbsp of maple syrup or agave

Steps:

1. In a saucepan, combine nondairy milk, water, and quinoa. Bring to a boil.
2. Reduce heat to medium-low, cover and cook for 15 minutes.
3. Remove from heat and let sit for 5 minutes.
4. Stir in cinnamon, nuts/seeds, and maple syrup or agave.

Nutrition Corner:

Calories: 145 | Carbs: 28 g | Protein: 5 g | Fat: 2.3 g | Sodium: 170 mg

2.17. Anti-Inflammatory Quinoa Fruit Bowl

Ready In:
Prep: 5 Min.
Assembly:5 Min.
Yields: 2 Soothing Bowls

What You'll Need:

- 1 - 1/2 cups cooked quinoa
- 3/4 cup unsweetened almond milk
- 1 banana, sliced
- 1/2 cup of cherries
- 1/2 cup of blueberries
- ¼ cup chopped walnuts
- 1 tablespoon turmeric-infused maple syrup

Steps:

1. Warm up the quinoa if it has cooled.

2. Layer each bowl equally starting with quinoa, followed by almond milk, banana slices, cherries, and blueberries.

3. Garnish with chopped walnuts.

4. Drizzle the turmeric-infused maple syrup over the top for a sweet anti-inflammatory touch.

Nutrition Facts:

Calories: 270 | Carbs: 48 g | Protein: 8 g | Fat: 8 g | Sodium: 45 mg

Chapter 3: Poultry and Meat Recipes

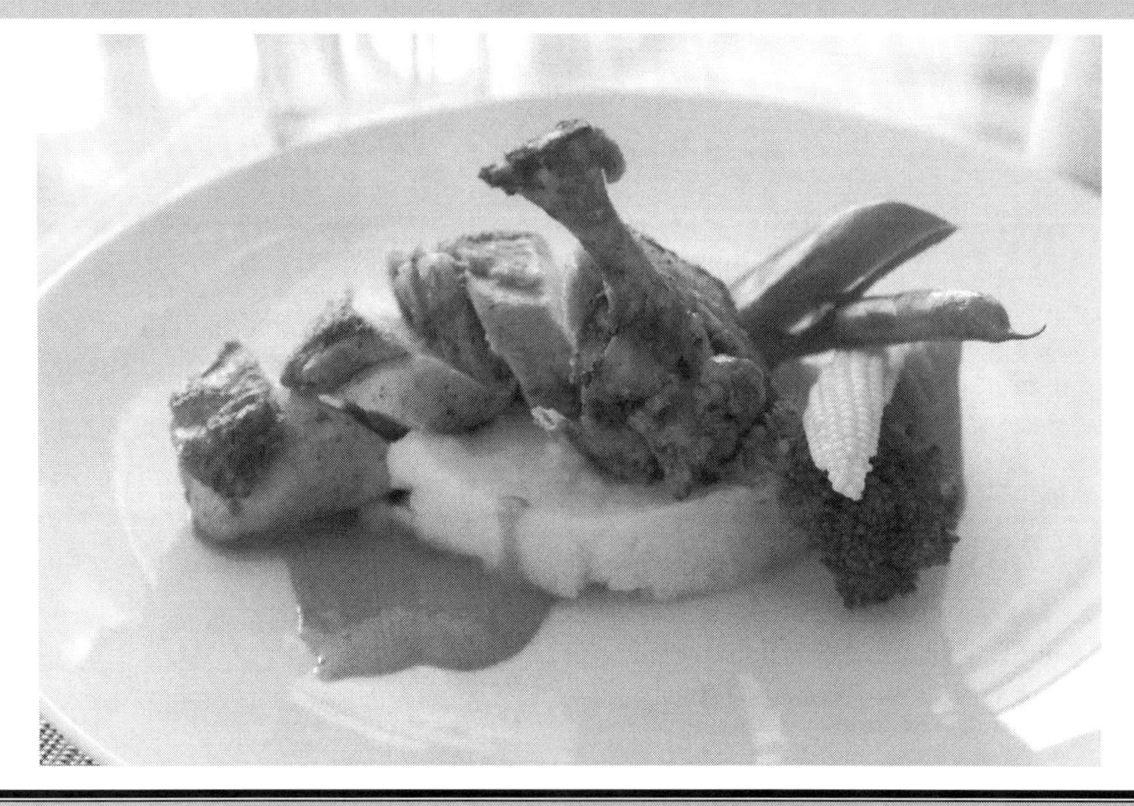

3.1. Crunchy Chicken Salad

Ready In:

- Prep: 10 Min.
- Cook: None, Just Chilling
- Serving: 6

What You'll Need:

- 2 cups cooked chicken
- 1 large hard-boiled egg, finely chopped
- 1/4 cup low-fat mayonnaise
- 2 tablespoons onion, minced
- 1/4 cup celery, diced
- A splash of lemon juice (about 1 teaspoon)
- A tiny sprinkle of sugar or Splenda (about 1/3 teaspoon)
- A dash of pepper

Instructions:

1. Start by tossing together your chicken, egg, onion, and celery in a generous-sized bowl.
2. In a separate, smaller bowl, whisk together the mayonnaise, lemon juice, your choice of sweetener, and pepper until smooth.
3. Marry the two mixtures, gently stirring until everything is beautifully coated.
4. Pop it in the fridge and let it chill. Giving it 2 hours or even overnight will make the flavors sing!
5. Ready to eat? Lay it on your favorite bread, roll, or pita. Add a leafy lettuce for some extra crunch if you're feeling it!

Nutritional Facts:

Calories: 125 | Carbs: 3 g | Protein: 167g | Fat: 18 g | Sodium: 96 mg

Heads-up: If you're keen on keeping inflammation at bay, consider swapping the sugar for a touch of honey or simply skipping it.

3.2. Anti-Inflammatory Blackened Chicken with Quail

Ready In:

- Prep: 5-7 Min.
- Cook: 15-20 Min.
- Serving: Feeds 6
-

What You'll Need:

- 3 chicken breasts and 6 quail
- 3 teaspoons olive oil and a bit more for brushing
- An anti-inflammatory spice blend:
- 3/4 tsp turmeric
- 1/2 tsp ginger powder
- 1/2 tsp paprika
- 1/3 tsp white pepper
- 1/3 tsp cumin
- 1/6 tsp garlic powder
- A pinch each of dried rosemary and salt

Instructions:

1. Preheat your oven to 350°F.
2. Combine all the spices in a mixing bowl to create your anti-inflammatory spice blend.
3. Gently brush the chicken breasts and quail with olive oil.
4. Then, generously season them with the spice blend, ensuring they are well-coated.
5. Using a pan heated on high,, quickly sear the chicken and quail – around 1 minute for quail and 1-2 minutes per side for chicken. They should attain a golden hue.
6. Transfer the chicken and quail to a baking sheet and roast in the oven. Quail will take about 8 minutes, while chicken will need about 12-15 minutes, or until cooked through.
7. Serve them up and enjoy the anti-inflammatory benefits!

Nutritional Facts:

Calories: 156; carbs: 1.5 g; protein: 48 g; fat: 6 g; sodium: 140 mg

3.3. Spicy Paprika Lamb Chops

Ready In:

- Prep: 10 Min-
- Cook: 10 Min.
- Serving: Enough For 4

What You'll Need:

- 0.5 lb. of luscious lamb racks, transformed into chops
- 1 tablespoon cumin powder (a bit less to keep things balanced)
- 3 tablespoons paprika
- 1 teaspoon chili powder
- Salt and pepper, seasoned to your liking

Instructions:

1. Get all those spices in a bowl and give them a good mix.
2. Rub this spicy concoction all over your lamb chops. Make sure every nook and cranny is seasoned.
3. Fire up the grill to a medium blaze.
4. Lay those chops down and let them sizzle. About 5 minutes on each side should get them to a juicy medium-rare.
5. Once they've got those perfect grill marks, plate them up. Enjoy the heat!

Nutritional Facts:

Calories: 490 | Carbs: 7 g | Protein: 100 g | Fat: 34 g | Sodium: 230 mg

3.4. Almond Chicken

Ready In:

- Prep.: 8 Min.
- Cook: 10-12 Min.
- Serving: Satisfies 3

What You'll Need:

- 2 chicken breasts, skinless and without bones
- half a lemon (squeezed)
- 1 and half cups of almond flour (it's like magic powder for chicken)
- 2 tablespoons of coconut oil
- Customized lemon pepper seasonin (homemade: add lemon peels to the black pepper)
- A sprinkle of parsley for that final flourish

Instructions:

1. Slice those chicken breasts in half, aiming for even 1/4-inch slices.
2. Dive them into the lemon juice for a quick dip, about 4 minutes, turning once.
3. Coat them in the almond meal – like you're tucking them into a crunchy blanket.
4. Melt the coconut oil in a pan over medium heat
5. Lay the chicken pieces in carefully.Let them cook for 4 minutes each side or until they're golden and tempting. As they cook, dust them with the lemon pepper.
6. Put them on a platter and garnish them with some chopped parsley. Voilà!

Nutritional Facts:

Calories: 360 | Carbs: 3 g | Protein: 44 g | Fat: 23 g | Sodium: 176 mg

3.5 Zesty Blackberry Chicken Wings

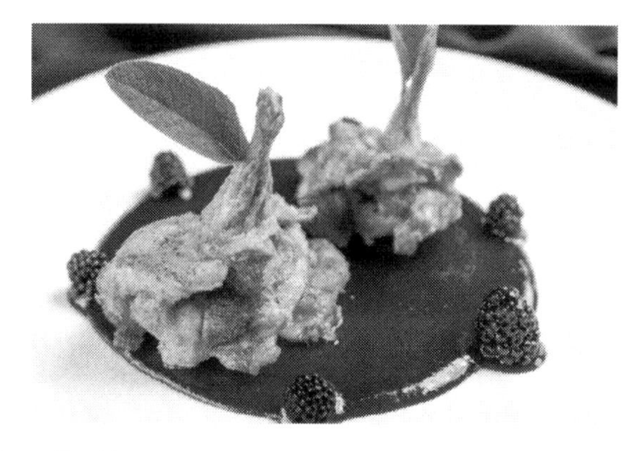

Ready In:

- Prep: 35 Min.
- Bake:45 Min.
- Serving: 2

What You'll Need:

- 0.75 pounds of chicken wings (about 20 pieces)
- 1/4 cup of blackberry-chipotle
- 1/4 cup of water
- Salt and freshly ground pepper to taste

Instructions

1. Begin with the marinade: Mix blackberry sauce and water in a bowl.
2. Save about a third of the marinade for later.
3. Place the wings in a zip bag, add the remaining marinade.
4. Salt and pepper them, then let them sit for 30 minutes.
5. Turn the oven on to 400°F.
6. Arrange the marinated wings on a baking sheet.
7. First bake: 15 minutes.
8. Brush them with the saved marinade.
9. Second bake: 30 minutes.
10. Serve and savor!

Nutritional Values

Calories: 702 | Carbohydrates: 1.8g | Protein: 45g | Fat: 29g | Sodium: 336mg

3.6 Toasted Sesame Grilled Chicken

Ready In:

- Prep :10 Min.
- Grill: 8 Min.
- Serving: 4

what you need:

- Vegetable cooking spray (preferably olive oil-based)
- 1 tablespoon toasted sesame seeds
- 1 tablespoon sherry
- 2 teaspoons grated ginger
- Four 4 oz. skinned chicken breast halves
- 1 tablespoon of choice sweetener (agave nectar or maple syrup)
- 1 tablespoon reduced-sodium soy sauce

Instructions

1. In a bowl, combine sesame seeds, sherry, ginger, sweetener, and soy sauce.
2. Flatten the chicken pieces to about ¼ inch thickness.
3. Spray your grill with the cooking spray.
4. For 4 minutes, grill the chicken on each side, brushing it regularly with the sauce.
5. Serve sprinkled with sesame seeds.

Nutritional Values

Calories: 179 | Carbohydrates: 11g | Protein: 27g | Fat: 3g | Sodium: 116mg

3.7 Dreamy Lemon-Tarragon Chicken

Ready In:

- Prep:5-8 Min.
- Cook: 15 Min.
- Serving: 4

what you need:

- Four boneless, skinless chicken breasts
- 1 cup fresh mushrooms (halved)
- 1/3 cup flour
- 2 cloves minced garlic
- 3 tablespoons dry sherry
- 1/2 teaspoon each of dried tarragon and lemon pepper seasoning
- 1 3/4 cups salt-free chicken broth
- 1/4 cup coconut cream
- 2 tablespoons of olive oil
- Your preferred noodles (whole grain or zucchini)

Instructions

1. In a pan on medium heat, warm the olive oil.
2. Add chicken, garlic, sherry, tarragon, mushrooms, and lemon pepper. Cook for about 10-12 minutes.
3. Set aside chicken and mushrooms.
4. Whisk together the chicken stock and flour, then add the mixture to the pan and stir until thickened.
5. Mix some sauce with the coconut cream, reintroduce chicken and mushrooms, warm but avoid boiling.
6. Serve over your choice of noodles.

Nutritional Values

Calories: 151 | Carbohydrates: 5g | Protein: 20g | Fat: 5g | Sodium: 96mg

3.8 Hearty Homestyle Meat Loaf

Ready In:

- Prep:10 Min.
- Bake:1 Hour 10 Min.
- Serving: 8

What You'll Need:

- 2 lightly beaten eggs
- 3/4 cup milk
- 2/3 cup breadcrumbs
- A pinch of sage
- 2 tablespoons finely chopped onions
- 1 1/2 lb. good quality ground beef
- 1/2 cup fresh mushroom slices

Topping

- 1/4 cup of shredded cheddar cheese
- 1/4 cup no-salt ketchup
- 1 teaspoon dry mustard
- 2 tablespoons brown sugar
- A hint of nutmeg

Instructions

1. In a big bowl, mix all the meatloaf ingredients together.
2. Make a loaf out of the mixture and place it in a loaf pan.
3. Warm up your oven to 350°F and slide in the pan.
4. After 1 hour, drain off any fat.
5. For that delicious topping, stir together the ketchup, mustard, sugar, and nutmeg. Spread this mix over your loaf. Finish with a sprinkle of cheese on top.
6. Put it back in the oven until the cheese melts just right or to your taste.

Nutritional Values

Calories: 335 | Carbohydrates: 14g | Protein: 26g | Fat: 19g | Sodium: 136mg

3.9 Steak with a Tender Onion Embrace

Ready In:

- Prep: 10 Min
- Cook :1 Hour
- Serving: 8

What You'll Need:

- 1/4 cup flour
- A hint of freshly ground pepper
- 1 1/2 lb. juicy round steak
- 1 cup water
- 1 tablespoon vinegar
- 1 minced garlic clove
- 2 tablespoons oil (of your choice)
- 1 bay leaf
- 1/4 teaspoon dried thyme
- 3 medium onions, finely sliced

Instructions

1. Divide that steak into 8 even portions.
2. Rub in the flour and pepper.
3. Heat up some oil and get those steaks seared to a nice brown.
4. Mix water, vinegar, garlic, bay leaf and thyme in a pot and bring to boil
5. Add your steak, and blanket it with those sliced onions.
6. Cover it up, and let everything simmer and mingle for 1 hour.

Nutritional Values

Calories: 271 | Carbohydrates: 6g | Protein: 18g | Fat: 19g | Sodium: 136mg

3.10 Golden Oven-Crisped Chicken

Ready In:

- Prep:10 Min.
- Cook:24 Min.
- Serving: 14

What You'll Need:

- 1 3-lb chicken, cleaned and ready
- 1/2 cup flour
- 1/4 cup healthier coconut oil
- 1/4 cup butter
- 1 teaspoon paprika
- A sprinkle of pepper
- 1/2 teaspoon onion powder

Instructions

1. Get your oven hot and ready at 425°F.
2. While that's happening, wash your chicken and pat it dry.
3. Melt your coconut oil and butter in a baking dish in the oven.
4. Mix up your flour, paprika, pepper, and onion powder in a separate bowl.
5. Drench each chicken piece in this mix.
6. Place them in the dish with the melted mix.
7. Give them about 24 minutes in the oven, turning once, until they're a beautiful golden brown and super tender inside.

Nutritional Values Calories: 184 | Carbohydrates: 2g | Protein: 21g | Fat: 10g | Sodium: 136mg

3.11 Tender chicken in sweet and sour sauce

Ready In:

- Prep: 8 Min.
- Cook:7 Min.
- Serves: 6

what you need:

- 1/2 cup honey (we've swapped out the sugar to keep it natural)
- 2 tablespoons of that zesty orange marmalade
- 1/2 cup vinegar
- 1/4 cup margarine (or butter if you prefer)
- 1 fresh green pepper, chopped into thin slices
- A can of pineapple chunks (20 oz.) don't forget we need the juice too!
- 1 lb. of tender chicken breasts, no bones or skin, and diced into cute 1/2-inch cubes
- 1 onion, sliced into those dreamy thin rings
- 2 tablespoons cornstarch (to get the right consistency)
- 3 cups of fluffy white rice, already cooked

Instructions

1. First off, drain your pineapple chunks, but be sure to save 1/3 cup of the juice – we'll need it later.
2. In your favorite mixing bowl, combine the honey and cornstarch smoothly. Stir in the pineapple chunks, the juice we saved earlier, vinegar, and orange marmalade. Let's put this bowl aside for a moment.
3. Time for some action! In a wok or a big pan, melt your margarine over a medium flame. Toss in the chicken cubes and give them a good stir-fry until they're golden, about 5 minutes should do.
4. Sliced onion and green pepper should be added now. Let them cook and mingle for another 2 minutes.
5. Here comes the magic – pour in the pineapple mixture.Stir it every now and then while you wait for it to boil.
6. Once done, serve this delightful mix over a plate of warm white rice.An alternative to the dish is to replace the rice with quinoa.

Nutritional Facts: Calories: 433 | Carbs: 67g | Protein: 21g | Fats: 9g | Sodium: 212mg

3.12 Turkey Fajitas

Ready In:

- Prep: 10 Min. (Plus, Be Patient For A 4-Hour Marinade)
- Cook: 20 Min.
- Servings: 10

What you'll need:

- 1 lb. of juicy boneless turkey breast
- A pinch (1/4 teaspoon) of pepper
- 1 garlic clove, minced to perfection
- 1 cup of vibrant chopped tomatoes
- Fresh cilantro, 1 tablespoon, finely chopped
- 1 tablespoon of your go-to cooking oil
- 3 cups of fresh shredded lettuce
- A dash (1 teaspoon) of chili powder
- More cilantro! Another 2 tablespoons, chopped
- 1 tablespoon of red onion, diced small
- Just a touch (1/4 teaspoon) of minced garlic
- The zest of 2 tablespoons of lime juice
- 10 fluffy 7-inch flour tortillas
- 1/2 cup of light and tangy sour cream

Instructions:

1. First, give your turkey a good rub-down with the pepper, garlic, chili powder, lime juice, that lovely cilantro, and oil. Get into every corner and cranny, then chill it in the fridge for about 3 hours.
2. While waiting, create a fresh salsa by mixing the tomato, cilantro, onion, and garlic. Put it in the fridge for an hour to chill.
3. When you're set, broil the turkey about 6 inches from the heat. Each side needs about 10 minutes to become beautifully cooked.
4. Once done, make thin turkey strips.
5. Wrap your tortillas in foil and let them warm up in the oven for 8 minutes.
6. Now, the fun part – assemble! Wrap up the turkey, salsa, lettuce, and sour cream in the tortillas. Delicious!

Nutrition Facts:

Calories: 208 | Carbs: 19g | Protein: 13g | Fats: 17g | Sodium: 126mg

3.13 Chicken Fingers with a Honeyed Dip

Ready In:

- Prep: 15 Min.
- Cooking: 20 Min.
- Serves: 4

For the Chicken:

- 1 ½ teaspoon of earthy dried thyme
- ¼ teaspoon of pepper
- ¾ cup breadcrumbs for that crispy coat
- 2 tablespoons of lovely Parmesan cheese
- ¾ teaspoon each of garlic and onion powder
- 4 chicken breast halves, skinless and boneless, cut into strips
- ¼ cup of melted, unsalted margarine

For the Honey Dip:

- ½ cup of light mayonnaise
- ½ teaspoon of aromatic dried dill weed
- A sweet ¼ cup of liquid honey

Steps to Yumminess:

1. Start with the dip: Mix the mayonnaise, honey, and dill. Let it chill in the fridge for about 30 minutes.
2. Turn your oven up to 400°F.
3. In a bowl, create your chicken's perfect outer layer by combining breadcrumbs, pepper, Parmesan, thyme, garlic, and onion powder.
4. Dip each chicken strip into the melted margarine, then give it a breadcrumb bath. Make sure it's well-coated!

5. On an oiled oven rack placed over a baking tray, lay your chicken strips down. Bake for 10 minutes, then flip and bake for another 10 minutes, until they are golden and delicious.
6. Enjoy with your honey dip!

Nutrition Facts: Calories: 290 | Carbs: 15g | Protein: 28g | Fats: 30g | Sodium: 136mg

3.14. Homestyle Turkey Meatloaf

Ready In:

- ➢ Pre :15 Min.
- ➢ Cook:55 Min.
- ➢ Serving Size: 6

What you'll need:

- 1 ½ lb. turkey mince
- 1 tablespoon olive oil
- 1 bay leaf
- 1 onion, finely chopped
- ¼ cup red bell pepper, finely chopped
- 2 eggs, whisked
- 1 teaspoon dried thyme
- 2 tablespoons Worcestershire Sauce
- 1/3 cup breadcrumbs
- ¼ cup ketchup (low sodium)

Instructions:

1. Warm up your oven to 325 degrees Fahrenheit.
2. Heat olive oil in a skillet over medium heat. Add the bell bell pepper and onions, season with thyme and bay leaf. Stir occasionally till the onions get that see-through look, roughly 6-7 minutes. Remember to remove the bay leaf afterward!
3. In a bowl, mix the turkey, breadcrumbs, eggs, Worcestershire sauce, and the sautéed onion mixture. Gently place this mix into a loaf pan.
4. Pop it in the oven and bake until the meatloaf has a spring in its step and reaches an internal temp of 160 degrees Fahrenheit.
5. Serve with a dash of ketchup, however you like!

Nutritional Facts: Calories: 283 | Carbs: 11 g | Protein: 26 g | Fat: 28 g | Sodium: 196 mg

3.15. Classic Chicken and Dumplings

Ready In:

- ➢ Prep:15 Min.
- ➢ Cook:1 Hour 30 Min.
- ➢ Yields: 6

What you need:

- 2 ½ lb. whole chicken
- 2-liter water
- ½ teaspoon pepper
- 3 tablespoons shortening
- 2 cups flour
- ½ teaspoon baking soda
- ¾ cup buttermilk (unsalted)

Instructions:

1. In a big pot, place the chicken and water. Turn up the heat until it's bubbling joyfully. Simmer it down for about an hour.
2. Take the chicken, set it aside and let it cool for a minute Once it's cool enough to handle, pull apart the meat.
3. Skim any extra bits floating in the pot.
4. Put the chicken back in, season with pepper, and bring back the boil.
5. Meanwhile, in a bowl, combine the flour, baking soda, and shortening. You're aiming for a breadcrumb-like consistency. Pour the buttermilk into the bowl and mix until the dough is smooth.
6. Flour your workspace, gently knead the dough, then roll it out. Cut or pinch small pieces to form dumplings.
7. One by one, place these dumplings into the boiling pot. Simmer until they're soft and fully cooked, stirring now and then.
8. Serve warm and let the cozy vibes of this dish envelop you!
   Nutritional Facts: KCal: 430 | Carbs: 33 g | Protein: 20 g | Fat: 22 g | Sodium: 126 mg

3.16. Chicken and Veggie Soba Noodles

Ready In:

- Prep:10 Min.
- Cook:10 Min.
- Serving Size: 4

What you'll need:

- 6 ounces uncooked soba noodles
- 2 cups no-salt or low-sodium chicken broth
- 1 red bell pepper, cut into thin strips
- 1 cup thinly sliced carrots
- 2 cups green cabbage, chopped
- 1 cup thawed edamame beans
- 1 can of chicken without added salt, drained and rinsed
- 1 (5-ounce) can of chicken breasts without added salt.
- ½ cup Peanut Apple Sauce
- A splash of water, if needed

Instructions:

1. Start by heating the chicken broth in a large pot till it gets all bubbly.
2. Slide in the soba noodles, cabbage, bell pepper, and carrots for a gentle simmer.
3. Let them mingle for about 5-7 minutes until the noodles soften and veggies become tender.
4. Time to join the party - toss in the edamame, canned chicken, and that tasty Peanut Apple Sauce. Stir well , making sure each bite has some sauce. Add a little water if it seems too thick.
5. Dish it out while it's hot and savor every spoon!

Nutritional Facts:

Calories: 369 | Carbs: 44 g | Protein: 19 g | Fat: 22 g | Sodium: 286 mg

3.17. Sizzling Jerk Chicken with Cozy Rice and Veggies

Ready In:

- Prep:15 Min. + 3 Hours to Marinate
- Cook:20 Min.
- Yields: 6

What you'll need:

- 1 small red onion, roughly chopped
- 6 fresh scallions, white and green bits (chopped)
- 1 tablespoon ginger (minced)
- 2 habanero chili peppers, seeds out and chopped
- 2 garlic buds (minced)
- A dash of white vinegar or lemon juice
- A spoonful of brown sugar or honey
- 2 teaspoons fresh thyme
- 1 tablespoon coconut amino
- 1 tablespoon avocado oil
- A pinch each of ground allspice, salt, nutmeg, cinnamon, and black pepper
- Cooking spray (avocado or olive oil variety)
- 12 ounces boneless, skinless chicken thighs
- 3 cups mixed frozen veggies
- 3 cups fluffy brown rice, cooked

Instructions:

1. Let's get our flavor game on! In a blender, toss in the onion, scallions, habanero, vinegar, brown sugar, coconut amino, oil, ginger, garlic, thyme, and those aromatic spices. Whiz until it's all smooth and creamy.
2. Marinate the chicken thighs in this flavorful mix. Let them soak up all the goodness in the fridge for at least 3 hours. Overnight works best!
3. Fire up your grill to a medium-high. Spray the chicken and let them sizzle until they're perfectly cooked, hitting an internal temp of 165°F.
4. Meanwhile, get your brown rice fluffy as per its packet's wisdom and steam those colorful veggies.

5. Lay out your perfectly grilled chicken next to a heap of rice and veggies. Dive in!

Nutritional Facts: Cal.: 301 | Carbs: 47 g | Protein: 12 g | Fat: 19 g | Sodium: 86 mg

3.18. Hearty Chicken Stir-Fry

Ready In:

- Prep: 10 Min.
- Cook: 20 Min.
- Serving Size:2

What you'll need:

- 1/3 cup brown rice (which will yield about 1 cup when cooked)
- 1 tbsp coconut aminos
- 1 tbsp red pepper flakes
- 2 tsp honey
- 2 garlic cloves, finely chopped
- 2 tsp rice wine vinegar
- 1 tsp cornstarch (mix with 2 tsp water to dissolve)
- 4 oz chicken breast without bones, chopped into bite-sized pieces
- 1 tbsp sesame oil, divided
- 6 cups frozen stir-fry veggies

Instructions:

1. Begin by preparing the brown rice according to its packaging.
2. In a bowl, combine coconut aminos, red pepper flakes, honey, vinegar, the cornstarch solution, and garlic.
3. Heat half a tablespoon of sesame oil over medium-high heat in a large frying pan. Add the chicken and cook for about 4-76minutes, or until golden brown.
4. Pour in the remaining sesame oil and introduce the frozen veggies. Continue cooking for another 5-6 minutes until they become hot and soft.
5. To serve, place half a cup of brown rice on a plate and top with chicken and vegetables.

Nutritional Facts Cal.: 362| Carb.: 54 g| Protein: 18 g| Fat: 23 g| Sodium 136 mg

3.19. Delightful Turkey Flatbread Pizza

Ready In:

- Preparation - 4 Minutes,
- Cooking - 16 Minutes
- Serving Size: Makes 1 Pizza

What you'll need:

- 1 Astoria's Family Bakery lavish flatbread
- 1 tbsp tomato paste (preferably without added salt)
- 1 oz slices of turkey (choose low-sodium or unsalted)
- 1 large mushroom, finely sliced
- 1 tsp Italian seasoning
- 1 small zucchini, sliced thin
- 1 mini red bell pepper, also thinly sliced
- ½ cup fresh baby kale, roughly chopped
- 2 tbsp grated mozzarella (low-sodium variant)

Instructions:

1. Preheat your oven to 350°F and position the flatbread on a baking tray.
2. Spread a layer of tomato paste over the flatbread, then sprinkle over the Italian seasoning.
3. Arrange your turkey, mushrooms, zucchini, bell pepper, and baby kale artistically on top. Finish with a scattering of mozzarella cheese.
4. Bake until the cheese is all melted and the veggies are cooked to your liking, around 16 minutes.

Nutritional Facts Calories: 238| Carbohydrates: 31 g| Protein: 19.4 g| Fat: 4 g| Sodium 88 mg |

3.20. Spicy Turkey Burgers

Ready in - 30 minutes (Preparation - 10 minutes, Baking - 20 minutes)

Serving size: Makes 5 burgers

What you'll need:

- Cooking spray (preferably avocado or olive oil-based)
- 12 oz lean ground turkey
- 1 cup yellow onion, finely minced
- ¼ cup panko breadcrumbs
- 1 large egg
- 1 cup of zucchini, finely chopped
- 1 jalapeño pepper, seeds removed (chopped)
- 1 tsp red pepper flakes
- 2 medium Poblano peppers, halved lengthwise (no seeds)
- 5 tsp Low-Sodium Dijon Mustard (this is optional)
- 5 whole-wheat hamburger buns
- ½ tsp garlic powder
- 5 romaine lettuce leaves
- a pinch of ground black pepper

Instructions:

1. Warm up the oven to 400°F. Prep a baking sheet with a spray of cooking oil and a lining of foil.
2. In a big mixing bowl, blend the turkey with zucchini, onion, breadcrumbs, egg, jalapeno, red pepper flakes, black pepper, and garlic powder.
3. With the dough, prepare five identical patties.
4. Lay out both patties and Poblano peppers on the prepped baking sheet.
5. Allow them to bake for 20-25 minutes or until the patties reach a temperature of 167°F on the inside.
6. Construct your burger! On the bottom half of a bun, spread mustard, add a lettuce leaf, a turkey patty, and a piece of Poblano pepper. Complete with the top half of the bun.
7. Enjoy immediately or keep the patties refrigerated for up to 5 days. For longer storage, layer patties with parchment paper in a sealed container and freeze.

Nutritional Facts Calories: 279| Carbohydrates: 24 g| Protein: 23 g| Fat: 10 g| Sodium 216 mg

3.21. Turkey Nuggets with Roasted Vegetables

Ready in:

- 35 minutes (Preparation - 10 minutes, Roasting - 25 minutes)
- Serving size: Makes 2 servings

What you'll need:

- 1 small zucchini, sliced into long strips
- 1 small broccoli bunch
- 1 medium carrot, also in long strips
- 1 small leek, again in long strips
- 1 medium-sized red bell pepper, sliced lengthwise into strips
- ½ of a small eggplant, in long strips
- 8 asparagus stalks, ends trimmed
- Cooking spray (avocado or olive oil variant)
- ¼ cup whole-grain panko bread crumbs
- 1 tbsp olive or avocado oil, split into two
- 5 oz turkey breast without skin or bones, cut into nugget-sized pieces
- 1 tsp Italian seasoning
- ½ cup brown lentils, cooked (if using canned, rinse and drain)

Instructions:

1. Put baking paper on a baking sheet and preheat the oven to 400°F.
2. Neatly arrange the veggies (zucchini, carrot, leek, bell pepper, eggplant, broccoli, and asparagus) on the baking sheet. Give them a light misting with the cooking spray.

3. Let them roast for around 25 minutes until they're golden and tender.
4. Meanwhile, in a bowl, stir together breadcrumbs, Italian seasoning, and half of your oil. Toss the turkey pieces in this mix until well coated.
5. In a pan over medium-high heat, heat the rest of the oil. Fry the turkey croquettes until they are fully cooked and reach golden brown.
6. For serving, mix half of the roasted veggies, half of the turkey nuggets, and lentils in a bowl.
7. It's best served hot, but any leftovers can be refrigerated up to 5 days.

Nutritional Facts

Calories: 287| Carbohydrates: 22 g| Protein: 18 g| Fat: 21 g| Sodium 296 mg

3.22. Turkey-Stuffed Bell Peppers

Ready in :

- 30 minutes (Preparation - 10 minutes, Cooking - 20 minutes)
- Serving size: Makes 4 stuffed peppers

What you'll need:

- 1 tbsp avocado oil
- 8 oz lean turkey mince
- ½ cup yellow onion, finely diced
- 1 cup carrots, grated
- ½ tsp garlic powder
- ½ tsp Italian seasoning mix
- 1 cup marinara sauce (no salt added)
- 4 bell peppers (you choose the colors!), tops removed, and seeds cleaned out

Instructions:

1. Warm the avocado oil in a large skillet over medium-high heat. Place the turkey, carrots and onion in the pot. Stir the turkey until cooked through.
2. Add the garlic powder, Italian spices and salsa. Let the ingredients cook together for 5/7 minutes.
3. Put all of this into the four peppers, stuffing them all the way to the top.
4. Steam or microwave these stuffed peppers until they're tender.
5. Serve hot!

Nutritional Facts

Calories: 307| Carbohydrates: 32 g| Protein: 19 g| Fat: 11 g| Sodium 86 mg

Chapter 4: Soup Recipes

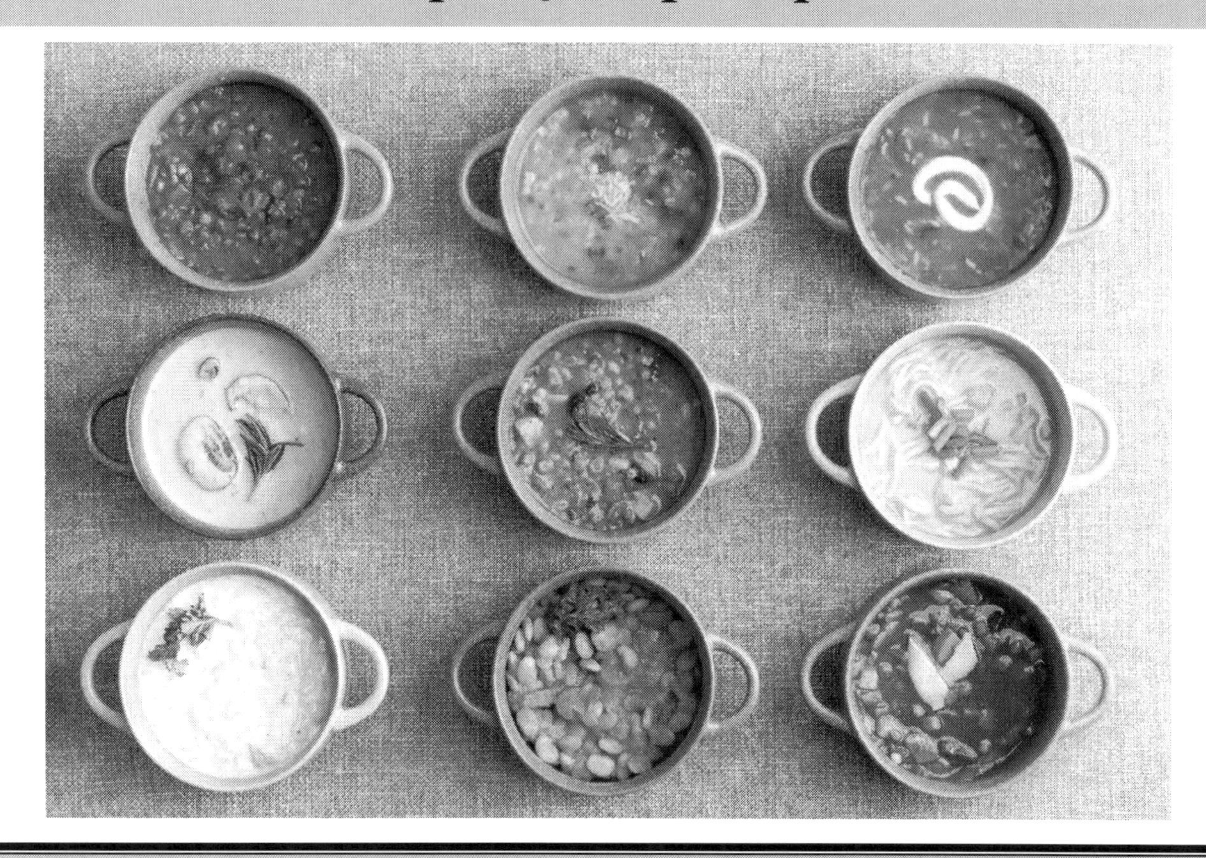

4.1. Eggplant Vegetable Soup

Ready In:

- Prep.: 8 Minutes
- Cook: 40 Min
- Serving: 12

What you need:

- 1/2 cup onion(chopped)
- 1 clove minced garlic
- 1/2 cup celery (chopped)
- 1/2 cup carrots (chopped)
- 1 lb 93% lean ground turkey
- 1 1/2 tsp ground nutmeg
- 1 can no-salt-added crushed tomatoes
- 1 medium eggplant, peeled and cubed
- 28 oz no-salt-added beef broth
- a pinch of salt
- 2 tsp dried parsley
- 1/2 cup dry macaroni
- 3/4 cup grated Parmesan cheese for garnish
- Pepper to taste

Directions:

1. In a pot, brown the turkey.
2. Add in onions, celery, carrots, tomatoes, and broth. Mix everything well.
3. Stir in the eggplant and seasonings, then let it simmer for 30 minutes.
4. Add the macaroni and cook for ten more minutes, or until the macaroni is cooked.
5. Add chopped parsley and stir.
6. Serve hot with a sprinkling of Parmesan cheese.

Nutritional Facts:

Calories 145 | Carbohydrates 12g | Proteins 13g | Fats 5.6g | Sodium 252mg

4.2. Turkey Vegetable Soup

Ready In:

- Prep.: 5 Min.| Cook: 15-20 Min.|
- Serving: 12

What you need:

- 1/4 cup unsalted butter
- 1 1/2 tsp low-sodium curry powder
- 2 tbsp flour
- 2 medium onions, shredded
- 1 cup chopped potatoes
- 1/2 cup celery (shredded)
- 1/2 cup carrots (shredded)
- 2 tbsp fresh parsley (shredded)
- 1/2 tsp fresh sage, shredded
- 3 cups low-sodium chicken broth
- 2 lb cooked 93% lean ground turkey
- 1/2 cups milk
- 10 oz frozen chopped spinach
- Pepper to taste

Instructions:

1 Melt the butter in a saucepan over medium-high heat. Sauté the onions in a skillet for about10 minutes or until they become translucent
2 Add the flour and curry powder, stirring well for 2-3 minutes.
3 Toss in potatoes, carrots, celery, parsley, and sage. Chicken broth should be added and the pot brought to a boil.
4 Cover and simmer on low heat for 10 minutes.
5 Combine the milk, spinach, and turkey. To heat everything evenly, stir and simmer for a few minutes.
6 To taste, add salt and pepper.

Nutritional Facts:

Cal. 245 | Carb. 8g | Proteins 24g | Fats 13.8g | Sodium 125mg

4.3. Ginger Pork Soup

Ready In:

- Prep.: 8 Min.| Cook: 20 Min.|
- Serving: 8

What you need:

- 1 tbsp olive oil
- 2 cups sliced shiitake mushrooms
- 12 oz lean boneless pork, thinly sliced
- 2 cloves garlic (minced)
- 32 oz low-sodium chicken broth
- 2 tsp fresh ginger
- 2 tbsp dry sherry
- 2 tbsp of low-sodium soy sauce
- 1/2 tsp of crushed red pepper
- 2 cups thinly sliced Chinese cabbage
- 1 scallion, thinly sliced

Instructions:

1 In a pot, heat the olive oil over medium heat. The pork should be cooked for about two minutes more until it is barely pink in the center. Set the pork aside.
2 In the same pot, sauté the garlic and mushrooms until soft.
3 Add the soy sauce, ginger, sherry, chili and chicken broth and bring to a boil.
4 Add back the pork, together with the green onion and Chinese cabbage.
5 Allow it to percolate until everything is thoroughly heated.

Nutritional Facts:

Calories 140 | Carbohydrates 8g | Proteins 13g | Fats 6.0g | Sodium 194mg

4.4. Creamy Thyme Carrot Soup

Ready In:

- Prep.: 12 Minutes| Cook: 25 Min.
- Serving: 12

Wat you need:

- cups low-salt vegetable or chicken broth
- 3 lbs baby carrots or carrot chunks (peeled)
- 1/2 tsp of ground ginger
- 1/3 cup honey
- 1/3 cup heavy cream
- 2 sprigs of fresh thyme
- Pepper to taste

Instructions:

1. In a large saucepan, bring together the carrots, broth, thyme.
2. When the boil is reached, lower the heat and allow to simmer for about 25 min. or until the carrots become tender.
3. When the soup is ready, remove it from the heat. Then remove the thyme sprigs and with an immersion blender, puree the soup until completely smooth.
4. Return the pureed soup to the original pot. Combine the cream and honey Stir well and season with ground ginger and pepper.
5. Reheat on a low flame if needed, then serve piping hot.

Nutritional Facts:

Cal. 100 | Carb. 17 g | Proteins 3 g | Fat 2.6 g | Sodium 433 mg

4.5. Cream of Corn Soup

Ready In:

- Prep.:15 Min.| Cook: 15 Min.
- Serving: 3

What you need:

- 2 tbsp melted margarine
- 2 tbsp flour
- 1/4 tsp pepper
- 1 quart of water
- 1 cup non-dairy creamer liquid
- Two jars (128 g each) of maize baby food in a strained cream style

Instructions:

1. In a medium-sized pot, melt the margarine.
2. Add the flour and pepper,, ensuring a smooth mix.
3. Gradually pour in the water and non-dairy creamer, continually stirring to avoid lumps.
4. The mixture should be brought to a boil, then reduce the heat
5. Stir in the corn baby food and let it simmer for a few minutes till it's heated through.

Nutritional Facts:

Calories 245 | Carbohydrates 22g | Protein 3g | Fat 16g | Sodium 164 mg

4.6. Cream of Crab Soup

Ready In:

- Prep.: 8 Min.| Cook: 20 Min.
- Serving: Four

Wat you need:

- 1 tbsp unsalted margarine
- 1/2 medium onion, finely chopped
- 1/2 lb shredded imitation crabmeat
- 1 quart low-sodium chicken broth
- 1 cup non-dairy coffee creamer
- 2 tbsp cornstarch
- 1/4 tsp dill weed

Instructions:

1. In a deep pot, melt the margarine over medium heat.
2. Add and sauté the onions
3. Cook for about 3 minutes after adding the crabmeat and stirring thoroughly.
4. Bring the mixture to a simmer with the chicken broth.
5. In a separate dish, whisk together the cornstarch and creamed milk until smooth.
6. Add this mixture to the saucepan gradually, stirring constantly, until the soup thickens.
7. Finish off with the dill weed, mix well, and serve while hot.

Nutritional Facts:

Calories 87 | Carbohydrates 7g | Protein 4g | Fat 5g | Sodium 241 mg

4.7 Rice and Chicken Soup

Ready In:

- Prep.:10 Min.| Cook: 40 Min.
- Servings: 3

What you need:

- 1 cup onions (chopped)
- 1 cup celery, sliced
- 3/4 cup uncooked white rice
- 1 cup carrots, chopped
- 1/2 tsp dried thyme leaves
- 1 leaf of bay
- 10 cups chicken broth (low salt)
- 2 boneless, skinless chicken breasts, cubed
- 1/2 tsp pepper
- 1/4 cup parsley, chopped
- 2 tbsp lime juice

Instructions:

1. Combine onions, celery, carrots, rice, pepper, thyme, bay leaf, and chicken broth in a sizable saucepan.
2. Bring to a gentle boil while stirring occasionally.
3. Cover, reduce heat to medium, and let it cook for twenty minutes.
4. Add the chicken cubes and cook for another 10 minutes uncovered.
5. Discard the bay leaf.
6. Before serving, incorporate the parsley and lime juice.

Nutritional Facts:

Calories 202 | Carbohydrates 22g | Protein 14g | Fats 6g | Sodium 52 mg

4.8 Soup with Carrot, Potato, and Leek

Ready In:

- Prep: 10 Min.|Cook: 20 Min. (10 Minutes for Boiling Vegetables)
- Servings: 4

Wat you need:

- 1 leek, chopped and cleaned
- 3/4 cup boiled potatoes, chopped
- 3/4 cup boiled carrots, diced
- 3/4 cup of uncooked white rice
- 1 garlic clove
- 1 tbsp canola oil
- Pepper to taste
- 3 cups low-sodium chicken broth
- 1/4 tsp cumin
- 1 bay leaf
- Parsley, chopped for garnish

Instructions:

1 Clean the leek by removing the tougher green parts. Slice thinly and rinse well in cold water, then drain.
2 In a sturdy saucepan, heat the oil.
3 For about 4 minutes, or until softened, sauté the leek and garlic over medium heat.
4 Add the cumin, pepper and bay leaf after pouring in the broth.
5 Stirring occasionally, bring the mixture to a boil over low heat.
6 Once the potatoes and carrots are cooked, add them to the mixture and continue simmering for another 10-15 minutes.
7 Discard the bay leaf, adjust seasoning, and serve sprinkled with chopped parsley.

Nutritional Facts:

Calories 92 | Carbohydrates 10g | Protein 4g | Fats 4g | Sodium 1084 mg

4.9 Roasted Red Pepper Soup

Ready In:

- Prep: 10 Min. Cook: 40 Min.
- Yields: 6

What you need

- 1/2 cup of roasted red peppers, shredded (around 3 peppers)
- 1 cup medium onions, thinly sliced (about 2 onions)
- 3 tbsp lemon juice
- 4 cups low-sodium chicken broth
- 1 tbsp fresh lemon zest, finely chopped
- 1 tsp cayenne pepper
- 1/4 tsp cinnamon
- 1/2 cup fresh cilantro, minced

Instructions:

1 Preheat your oven to 400°F. Roast the peppers on a baking sheet covered in parchment paper for 20 minutes, rotating once halfway through cooking, until tender.
2 Let the peppers cool for 5 minutes. Once cooled, peel off their skins, remove the seeds and slice them thinly.
3 In a medium stockpot, combine all the ingredients except for the cilantro.
4 The mixture should be brought to a boil over high heat before being reduced to a simmer. Allow the soup to simmer, partially covered, for approximately 15 minutes, or until it has thickened somewhat.
5 The soup needs to cool down a little. Put in a blender or use a hand blender to mix until smooth.
6 Return to heat and stir in the cilantro. Serve warm.

Nutritional Facts:

Calories 91 | Carbohydrates 15g | Protein 5g | Fats 6g | Sodium 676 mg

4.10. French Onion Soup

Ready In:

- Prep: 18 Min.| Cook: 35 Min.
- Yields: 4

What you need

- 4 sliced Vidalia onions
- 2 cups low-sodium chicken broth
- 2 tbsp butter (unsalted)
- 2 cups water
- 1 tbsp fresh thyme, chopped
- Black pepper, to taste

Instructions

1. In a large pot, melt the butter over medium heat.
2. Toss in the onions and cook them down for 20 minutes, or until they're golden and caramelized. Keep from burning by stirring every so often.
3. Add the water and chicken broth and bring to a boil.
4. Reduce the heat, add the thyme, and simmer for another 10 minutes.
5. Season with black pepper to taste.
6. Serve hot.

Nutritional Facts

Calories 90 | Carbohydrates 7g | Protein 2g | Fats 3g | Sodium 57 mg

4.11. Cream of Watercress Soup

Ready In:

- Prep: 25 Min. | Cook: 40 Min.
- Yields: 4

What you need:

- 1/2 tablespoon olive oil
- 1 noice of unsalted butter
- 1/2 oz chopped onion
- 1 tablespoon lemon juice
- 4 cups watercress, chopped
- cloves of garlic
- 1/2 tablespoon olive oil
- 1 noice of unsalted butter
- 1/2 oz chopped onion
- 4 cups watercress, chopped
- 1/4 cup chopped parsley
- 3 quarts of water
- 1/4 cup heavy cream
- Black pepper, to taste

Instructions:

1 Preheat the oven to 375°F.
2 Wrap the garlic in a foil bag after placing the cloves on the sheet and drizzling with olive oil.
3 Roast for 20 minutes or until softened. Once cooled, squeeze out the roasted garlic pulp.
4 Melt the butter in a large saucepan over low heat.
5 Add onions and sauté until translucent, around 2-5 minutes.
6 Add the watercress and parsley, continuing to sauté for another 5 minutes.
7 Add the roasted garlic pulp and water and stir. To cook the veggies, bring the mixture to a boil, then decrease the heat and simmer for 20 minutes.
8 Take it off the stove and let it cool down a bit. You may use a hand blender or work in batches in a food processor to puree the soup.
9 Bring the soup back to a simmer and stir in the heavy cream. Warm it up, add some lemon juice, and season it with black pepper.

Nutritional Facts

Calories 97 | Carbohydrates 5g | Protein 2g | Fats 8g | Sodium 23 mg

4.12. Mesmerizing Lentil Soup

Ready In:

- Prep.: 8 Min. (Plus Soaking Time) Cook: 8 Hours
- Yields: 4

What you need

- 1 lb dried lentils, soaked overnight and rinsed
- 3 carrots, peeled and chopped
- 1 celery stalk, chopped
- 1 onion, chopped
- cups low-sodium vegetable broth
- 1 ½ tsp of garlic powder
- 1 tsp ground cumin
- 1 tsp of smoked paprika
- 1 tsp dried thyme
- ¼ tsp liquid smoke
- ¼ tsp ground pepper

Instructions

1 Add all ingredients to a slow cooker, stirring to combine.
2 Cover and simmer on low heat for eight hours.
3 Before serving, give it a good stir and adjust seasoning if necessary.

Nutritional Facts

Calories: 307 | Fat: 1g | Carbohydrates 56g | Protein 20g | Sodium 145 mg

4.13. Cream of Mushroom Soup

Ready In:

- Prep: 10 Min.| Cook: 20 Min.
- Yields: 5

What you need

- 220 g(8 ounce) fresh mushrooms
- ¼ cup onion, chopped
- 2 tablespoons unsalted butter
- 2 cans of reduced-sodium chicken broth
- tablespoons whole-wheat flour
- half cup of cream
- half cup fat-free cream
- A pinch of salt and pepper

Instructions

1 In a large saucepan, melt the butter over medium heat. The onion and mushrooms should be added and cooked until soft.
2 In a separate bowl, whisk together the flour, salt, pepper, and one can of chicken broth until smooth.
3 Add the mushrooms to the flour mixture , pour them into the saucepan and stir everything together
4 Add the rest of the broth and bring the soup to a boil. Prepare for about 2 to 3 minutes, or until thickened.
5 Lower the flame, stir the cream, and simmer for another 10 minutes, allowing flavors to meld.

Nutritional Facts

Calories 74 | Carbohydrate 9.8g | Protein 6g | Fat 9.4g | Sodium 129 mg

4.14. Roasted Vegetable Soup

Ready In:

- Prep: 15 Min.| Cook: 20 Min.
- Yields: 2

What you need

- 1 tbsp olive oil
- garlic cloves, peeled
- 0.3 lb potatoes, diced (1 cm thick)
- 2 bell peppers, diced
- ½ tsp fresh rosemary, finely chopped
- 1 carrot, halved lengthwise (cut into 1 cm pieces)
- 1 tsp fresh tarragon
- 1 red onion, in chunks
- 0.4 qt carrot juice
- 0.3 lb of Italian tomatoes, diced
- A pinch of pepper and salt

Instructions:

1 Bring the oven to 400° F.
2 On a baking tray, combine potatoes, peppers, garlic, carrot, onion, and tomatoes. Drizzle with olive oil Roast for 10 to 15 minutes after being drizzled with olive oil.
3 and roast for 10-15 minutes. Put the carrot juice and tarragon in a saucepan and heat until the liquid boils.
4 Incorporate the roasted vegetables and mix well. Simmer briefly. Season with salt, pepper, and rosemary. Serve warm.

Nutritional Facts:

Calories 318 | Carbohydrates 60g | Protein 1.7g | Fat 9.7g | Sodium 40mg

4.15. Creamy Asparagus Soup

Ready In:

- Prep: 15 Min.| Cook: 25 Min.
- Yields: 4

What you need:

- stems of white asparagus
- Pinch sugar
- 2 tbsp olive oil
- 2 tbsp flour
- 1 egg yolk
- 1 tsp of fresh lemon juice
- stems leaf parsley
- 1.5-2L Water
- Pinch of salt

Instructions:

1 Thoroughly peel the asparagus. Remove 2 cm from the woody end and slice the asparagus diagonally into 2 cm segments.
2 Add asparagus, water, salt and a pinch of sugar to a saucepan and bring to a boil. For 15 minutes, simmer once the water has come to a boil.
3 Transfer asparagus broth to a new pot and bring to a boil again, leaving the asparagus pieces for 5-7 minutes.
4 Remove and set aside. In another pot, heat olive oil and mix in the flour. Whisk in 1L of asparagus broth.
5 Remove from heat and gently mix in egg yolk. Blend until smooth, return asparagus pieces to the soup, and heat briefly.
6 Garnish with freshly chopped parsley before serving.

Nutritional Facts:

Calories 126 | Carbohydrates 12.1g | Protein 6.2g | Fat 7.4g | Sodium 251mg

4.16. Curried Cauliflower Soup

Ready In:

- Prep: 20 Min.| Cook: 20 Min.
- Yields: 6

What you need:

- 2 tsp garlic, minced
- 1 cauliflower head, chopped into tiny florets
- cups water
- 1 tablespoons olive oil
- 2 tbsp curry powder
- 1/2 cup coconut yogurt
- 1 sweet onion, sliced
- 3 tablespoons of chopped parsley

Instructions:

1 To soften the onion and garlic,
2 Sauté the two ingredients in the olive oil over medium heat.. Curry powder, water, and cauliflower should be added. Cauliflower should be cooked until soft, so bring to a boil and then simmer.
3 Put the soup in a blender and process until smooth. Stir in some coconut yogurt and fresh cilantro and return to the saucepan.
4 Warm over medium-low heat for 5 minutes.

Nutritional Facts: Calories 83 | Carbohydrates 11g | Protein 3g | Fats 3.7g | Sodium 27mg

4.17. Soup with eggplant and red peppers

Ready In:

- Prep: 15 Min.| Cook: 20 Min.
- Yields: 6

What you need:

- 1 quartered tiny, sweet onion
- 2 halved tiny red bell peppers
- 1 tablespoon olive oil
- 2 cups eggplant cubes
- 2 smashed garlic cloves
- 1 cup chicken stock (easy) (here)
- 14 cup fresh basil, chopped
- Black pepper, freshly ground

Instructions

1 Oven and preheat to 350 degrees Fahrenheit. Combine the onions, red peppers, eggplant, and garlic in a large baking dish. Drizzle the olive oil over the veggies. Toast for 30 minutes, or until vegetables are soft and have a faint browned color.
2 Allow the veggies to cool somewhat before peeling the peppers. Purée the veggies with the chicken stock in stages in a blender (or a large mixing container with a handheld immersion blender).
3 Transmit the soup to a big pan and add just enough water to thin it down to your desired consistency.
4 Take the soup to a low boil and stir in the basil. Serve with a pinch of black pepper.

Nutritional Facts

Calories 61| Carbohydrates 9g| Protein 2g| Fats 2g| Sodium 95 mg |

4.18. Turkey Bulgur Soup

Ready In:

- Prep: 25 Min.| Cook: 22 Min.
- Yields: 6

What you need:

- 1 teaspoon of extra virgin olive oil
- 1/2-pound cooked ground turkey (93% thin)
- 1/2 oz. sweet onion (chopped)
- 1 teaspoon of garlic, crushed
- 1 cup of chicken stock
- 1 chopped celery stalk
- 1 thinly sliced carrot
- 1/2 cup of green cabbage, shredded
- 1/2 cup of bulgur 2 bay leaves, dry
- 2 tablespoons of parsley, chopped
- 1 teaspoon of fresh sage, chopped
- 1 teaspoon thyme, diced
- 1 tablespoon red pepper pinches
- Four cups water
- Pepper for taste

Instructions

1 Heat the oil in a large saucepan or frying pan over medium-high heat.
2 Cook until the turkey is cooked through.
3 Add the onion and garlic and sauté for three minutes, or until the vegetables are tender. Celery, carrot, cabbage, bulgur, and bay leaves should be added to the water, chicken stock, celery, carrot, cabbage, and bulgur.
4 Carry the soup to boiling, reduce the heat to low, and stew for 35 minutes, or until the bulgur or vegetables are soft.
5 With the bay leaves gone, mix the parsley, sage, thyme, and red pepper flakes.
6 Serve with a pinch of black pepper.

Nutritional Facts

Calories 77|Carbohydrates 2g|Protein 8g|Fats 6g| Sodium 54 mg |

4.19. Ground Beef and Rice Soup

Ready In:

- Prep: 12 Min.| Cook: 25 Min.
- Yields: 6

What you need:

- 1/2 pound of beef (extra-lean)
- 1/2 onion, minced
- 1/2 teaspoon of garlic trimmed
- 2 cups of water
- 1/2 cup of green beans, divided into 1-inch pieces
- 1 teaspoon of thyme, shredded
- 1/2 cup of uncooked long-grain white rice
- Pepper

Instructions

1 Over medium-high heat, place the ground beef in a large pot or frying pan. Approximately 6 minutes, often stirring, or until the beef is well-browned.
2 Remove any remaining grease from the heat.
3 Stir the onion and garlic. Cook for another 3 minutes or till the veggies get softened. Meld the water, chicken bouillon, rice, and celery in a large mixing bowl.
4 Carry the soup to a boil, lower to low heat and cook for 30 minutes until the rice is softer. Simmer for 3 minutes with the green beans and thyme.
5 Season with pepper after removing the soup from the heat.

Nutritional Facts

Calories 154| Carbohydrates 14g| Protein 9g|Fats 7g| Sodium 133 mg

Chapter 5: Vegetable Recipes

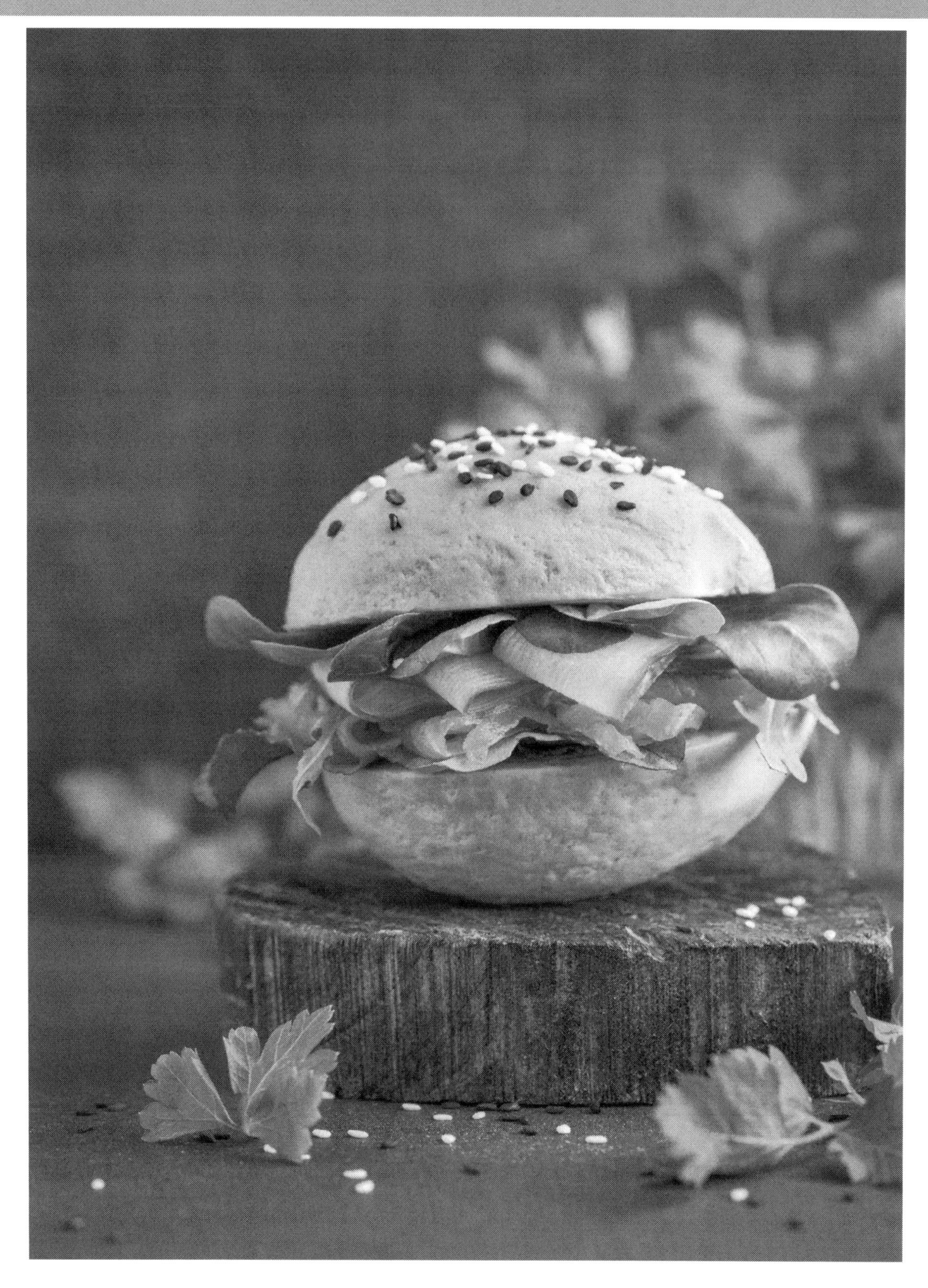

5.1. Healthy Golden Eggplant Fries

Ready In:

- Preparation-Baking Times: 10 Min. | 15 Min.
- Serving: 8

What you need:

- 2 eggs
- Sunflower seeds and pepper as required
- 2 cups almond flour
- 2 tbsp coconut oil (for spray)
- 2 eggplants (peeled and cut thinly)

Instructions:

1. Preheat your oven to 400 degrees Fahrenheit. In a mixing bowl, combine almond flour, sunflower seeds, and black pepper.
2. In a separate bowl, whisk the eggs until they become foamy. Dip the eggplant slices in the eggs, followed by the flour mixture.
3. Line a baking sheet with parchment paper and lightly spray with coconut oil. Place the coated eggplant slices on the sheet.
4. Reduce the oven temperature to 350°F and bake the eggplants for 15 minutes or until golden and crispy. Serve immediately and enjoy!

Nutritional Facts:

Calories: 855.72 | Carbohydrates: 42.55 g | Protein: 30.63 g | Fat: 69.01 g | Sodium 86 mg

5.2. Wild Mushroom Pilaf

Ready In:

- Preparation-Baking Times: 10 Minutes |30 Min.
- Serving: 4

What you need:

- 1 cup of wild rice
- 1/2-pound baby Bella mushrooms
- 2 cups water
- green onions (chopped)
- 2 garlic cloves (minced)
- 2 tbsp olive oil

Instructions:

1. In a large saucepan, heat the olive oil over medium heat.
2. Add the minced garlic and chopped green onions. Once the onions have turned translucent, add in the mushrooms and sauté for a few minutes until they're tender.
3. Stir in the wild rice, ensuring each grain gets coated with the oil mixture. Meanwhile, bring the 2 cups of water to a boil in a separate pot.
4. Pour the boiling water over the rice mixture, stirring constantly.
5. Reduce the heat to low, cover, and simmer for 30 minutes or until the rice is cooked through. Fluff with a fork, serve, and enjoy!

Nutritional Facts:

Calories: 210 | Carbohydrates: 16 g | Protein: 4 g | Fat: 6 g | Sodium 312 mg

5.3. Sporty Baby Carrots

Ready In:

- Preparation-Baking Times: 5 Min. | 7 Min.
- Serving: 4

What you need:

- 1-pound baby carrots
- 1 cup water
- 1 tbsp fresh mint leaves (chopped)
- 1 tbsp clarified ghee
- Sea flavored vinegar, to taste

Instructions:

1. In a pot, bring the water to a boil.
2. Add the baby carrots and blanch for about 2 minutes until they are slightly tender. Drain the water and set the carrots aside.
3. In the same pot, melt the clarified ghee and sauté the chopped mint leaves for 30 seconds.
4. Add the blanched carrots back into the pot and sauté for an additional 5 minutes until they are fully tender.
5. Drizzle with sea flavored vinegar to taste.

Nutritional Facts:

Calories: 131 | Carbohydrates: 11 g | Protein: 2 g | Fat: 10 g | Sodium 286 mg

5.4. Saucy Garlic Greens

Ready In:

- Preparation-Baking Times: 5 Minutes | 20 Minutes
- Serving: 4

What you need:

- 1/2 cup cashews
- 1/4 cup water
- 1 tbsp lemon juice
- 1 garlic clove (peeled)
- 1 tsp coconut amino
- 1/8 tsp flavored vinegar
- 1 bunch leafy greens

Instructions:

1. First, create the sauce by blending the soaked cashews (make sure you've drained the soaking water), fresh water, lemon juice, flavored vinegar, coconut amino, and garlic until you have a smooth, creamy consistency.
2. Transfer the sauce to a bowl and set aside. In a pot, add about 1/2 cup of water and bring it to a boil.
3. Add in the leafy greens and steam for about 1 minute. Drain the excess water and transfer the greens to a mixing bowl.
4. Pour over the prepared sauce and toss the greens until well coated.

Nutritional Facts:

Calories: 196 | Carbohydrates: 11.3 g | Protein: 5.25 g | Fat: 15.88 g | Sodium 176 mg

5.5. Pasta with Creamy Broccoli Sauce

Ready In:

- Preparation-Baking Times: 15-20 Minutes
- Serving: 2

What you need:

- 1 tbsp olive oil
- 0.25 lb broccoli florets
- 1.5 garlic cloves, halved
- 1/2 cup low-salt vegetable broth
- 1/4 cup whole-wheat spaghetti pasta
- 1/2 tsp dried basil leaves
- 2 tbsp cream cheese

Instructions:

1 Bring a pot of water to a boil and cook the pasta for 12-14 minutes or as per package instructions. Reserve a cup of pasta water and then drain.
2 Meanwhile, heat olive oil in a pan and sauté broccoli and garlic for 3 minutes.
3 Add vegetable broth to the pan and simmer on low heat for 5–6 minutes until broccoli softens.
4 In an immersion blender, combine the softened broccoli, cream cheese, and basil. Purée half the mixture until smooth and return it to the pan.
5 Mix the cooked pasta with the broccoli sauce, adding reserved pasta water as needed to coat the pasta evenly.
6 Serve hot and enjoy!

Nutritional Facts:

Color.: 410 | Carb.: 35g | Protein: 11g | Fat: 26g | Sodium: 286mg

5.6. Delicious Vegetarian Lasagna

Ready In:

- Preparation-Baking Times: 35 Minutes
- Serving: 4

What you need:

- 1 tsp basil
- 1 cup sliced eggplant
- 1/2 red pepper, sliced
- 2 lasagna sheets
- 1/4 tsp black pepper
- 1 cup rice milk
- 1/2 red onion, diced
- 1 garlic clove, minced
- 1/2 zucchini, sliced
- 1/2 pack soft tofu
- 1 tsp oregano
- 1 tbsp olive oil

Instructions:

1 Preheat your oven to 325°F.
2 Vertically slice the zucchini, eggplant, and pepper.
3 In a food processor, combine rice milk and tofu. Process until smooth.
4 In a pan, heat olive oil and sauté garlic and onions until tender.
5 Add oregano, black pepper, and basil. Continue to sauté for 5-6 minutes.
6 Layer an oven dish with a lasagna sheet, followed by 1/3 each of the eggplant, zucchini, pepper, and white tofu sauce. Repeat for the next two layers, finishing with the sauce.
7 Bake for 25 minutes or until the vegetables are tender.
8 Serve hot!

Nutritional Facts:

Calories: 235 | Carbohydrates: 10g | Protein: 5g | Fat: 9g | Sodium: 86mg

5.7. Pesto Pasta with Cream

Ready In:

- Preparation-Baking Times: 30 Minutes
- Serving: 4

What you need:

- oz linguine noodles
- 2 cups packed arugula leaves
- 2 cups packed basil leaves
- 1/3 cup walnut pieces
- tbsp extra-virgin olive oil
- 3 garlic cloves
- Freshly ground black pepper

Instructions:

1 Boil a pot of water and cook the linguine for 10-12 minutes until al dente. Drain.
2 In a food processor, combine basil, arugula, walnuts, and garlic. Process until coarsely ground.
3 Drizzle in the olive oil slowly, processing until the mixture is smooth.
4 Season with salt and black pepper.
5 Toss the drained linguine with the pesto sauce and serve immediately.

Nutritional Facts:

Calories: 394 | Carbohydrates: 40g | Protein: 10g | Fat: 21g | Sodium: 236mg

5.8. Garden Salad

Ready In:

- Preparation-Baking Times: 10 Minutes
- Serving: 4

What you need:

- oz raw peanuts in the shell
- 1 bay leaf
- 1 medium red bell pepper, chopped
- tbsp + 1 tsp green pepper, diced
- 0.5 tsp flavored vinegar
- tbsp +1 tsp sweet onion, diced
- 2 tbsp +2 tsp hot pepper, finely diced
- 2 tbsp + 2 tsp celery, diced
- 1 tbsp + 1 tsp olive oil
- ¼ tsp freshly ground black pepper

Instructions:

1 In a large salad bowl, combine the red bell pepper, green pepper, sweet onion, hot pepper, and celery.
2 In a small bowl, whisk together the olive oil, flavored vinegar, and black pepper to make a dressing.
3 Drizzle the dressing over the salad and toss to combine.
4 Garnish with raw peanuts and serve immediately.

Nutritional Facts:

Calories: 240 | Carbohydrates: 24g | Protein: 5g | Fat: 14g | Sodium: 136mg

5.9. Zucchini Pasta

Ready In:

- Prep 15 Min| Cook: 25 Min.
- Serving: 4

What you need:

- 1 1/2 cloves of garlic (minced)
- large zucchinis (diced)
- 1/2 cup 2% milk
- 1/4 tsp nutmeg
- 1 tbsp fresh lemon juice
- 1/2 cup grated cheddar
- oz uncooked farfalle pasta
- Sea salt and black pepper to taste
- tbsp olive oil

Instructions

1. In a skillet over medium heat, heat the olive oil. Add the minced garlic and cook for a minute, stirring frequently to prevent burning.
2. Season with salt and pepper.
3. Add the diced zucchini and stir thoroughly.
4. Cover and cook for about 15 minutes, stirring occasionally.
5. In a microwave-safe bowl, warm the milk for 30 seconds. Stir in the nutmeg to the milk and then add this mixture to the skillet. Cook uncovered for an additional 5 minutes, stirring occasionally.
6. Meanwhile, prepare the farfalle pasta in a stockpot as per the package instructions. Reserve two tablespoons of pasta water after draining.
7. To the skillet, add the cheese, lemon juice, and the reserved pasta water, stirring to combine.

Nutritional Facts

Calories: 813.76 | Carbs: 99.71g | Protein: 27.15g | Fat: 34.79g | Sodium: 136mg

5.10. Spicy Cabbage Dish

Ready In:

- Prep: 8 Min.| Cooking Time: 25-30 Min.
- Serving: 4

What you need:

- 2 yellow onions (chopped)
- cups red cabbage (shredded)
- 1 cup plums (pitted and chopped)
- 1 garlic clove (minced)
- 1 tsp cumin seeds
- 1 tsp coriander seeds
- 1 tsp cinnamon powder
- 1/4 tsp ground cloves
- 2 tbsp red wine vinegar
- 1/2 cup water

Instructions

1. In a slow cooker or large pot, combine the cabbage, garlic, cumin, coriander, water, onions, and other ingredients.
2. Stir to mix well.
3. Cabbage should be cooked for 20-30 minutes over low heat. Use separate plates for each person.

Nutritional Facts

Calories: 219.48 | Carbs: 51.05g | Protein: 3g | Fat: 1.38g | Sodium: 146mg

5.11. Peas Soup

Ready In:

- Prep: 8 Min.| Cook: 10 Min.
- Serving: 2

What you need:

- 1 egg
- 1 cup peas
- 1/2 chopped white onion
- 1/2-quart veggie stock
- 1 1/2 tbsp lemon juice
- 1 tbsp grated parmesan
- 1/2 tsp olive oil
- A pinch of salt
- Black pepper to taste

Instructions

1. In a saucepan over medium-high heat, heat the olive oil. Add the onions and cook until softened, about 4 minutes.
2. Add the peas, veggie stock, and lemon juice. Bring to a simmer and let it cook for 4 minutes.
3. Slowly stir in the whisked egg, letting it cook and thicken for Two minutes.
4. Season with salt, pepper, and parmesan.
5. Pour into bowls and serve.

Nutritional Facts

Calories: 264 | Carbs: 33g | Protein: 17g | Fat: 7.2g | Sodium: 126mg

5.12. Basil Zucchini Spaghetti

Ready In:

- Prep:1 Hour 10 Min.| Cook: 10 Min.Ù
- Serving: 4

What you need:

- 1/3 cup melted coconut oil
- zucchinis (spiralized)
- 1/4 cup chopped basil
- 1/4 cup chopped walnuts
- 2 garlic cloves (minced)
- Salt and pepper to taste

Instructions

1. In a bowl, combine spiralized zucchini with salt and pepper. Let it sit for 1 hour, then drain any excess water.
2. In a pan over medium-high heat, warm the coconut oil. Add the zucchini and garlic, stirring for about 5 minutes.
3. Mix in basil, walnuts, and season with black pepper. Continue cooking for 3 more minutes. Serve as a side dish.

Nutritional Facts

Calories: 287 | Carbs: 8g | Protein: 4g | Fat: 27g | Sodium: 186mg

5.13. Cauliflower Rice and Coconut

Ready In:

- Prep.: 20 Min.| Cook: 15-20 Min.
- Serving: 4

What you need:

- cups riced cauliflower
- 1-2 tsp sriracha paste
- 2/3 cup full-fat coconut milk
- 1/4- 1/2 tsp onion powder
- A pinch of salt
- Basil for garnish

Instructions

1 In a pan over medium-low heat, combine riced cauliflower, sriracha, coconut milk, and onion powder. Stir to combine.
2 Cover and cook for 6-10 minutes or until most of the liquid is absorbed.
3 Once the cauliflower rice is creamy and cooked through, adjust the seasoning. Serve garnished with fresh basil.

Nutritional Facts

Calories: 225 | Carbs: 4g | Protein: 5g | Fat: 19g | Sodium: 196mg

5.14. Kale and Garlic Platter

Ready In:

- Prep: 3 Min.| Cook: 12 Min.
- Serving: 2

What you need:

- ½ of bunch kale
- 1 tbsp of olive oil
- 2 garlic cloves (minced)

Instructions

1 Remove the stems from the kale and chop them into bite-sized pieces.
2 Heat the olive oil over medium heat in a large, heavy-bottomed saucepan.
3 Add the garlic and sauté for 2 minutes.
4 Add the kale and cook for 5-10 minutes, stirring occasionally.
5 Serve hot.

Nutritional Facts:

Calories: 121 | Carbohydrates: 6 g | Protein: 4 g | Fat: 8 g | Sodium: 129 mg

5.15. Blistered Beans and Almond

Ready In:

- Prep:10 Min. | Cook: 20 Min.
- Serving: 2

What you need:

- 1/2 lb fresh green beans (ends trimmed)
- 1 tbsp olive oil
- 1 tbsp fresh dill (minced)
- Juice of 1/2 lemon
- 1/8 cup crushed almonds
- 1/8 tsp salt
- Additional salt to taste

Instructions:

1 Preheat the oven to 400°F (200°C).
2 In a mixing bowl, toss the green beans with olive oil and 1/8 tsp salt.
3 Spread them on a large baking sheet.
4 Roast in the preheated oven for 10 minutes.
5 Stir the beans and roast for an additional 8-10 minutes or until blistered.
6 Remove from the oven and transfer to a mixing bowl.
7 Drizzle with lemon juice, sprinkle minced dill, and mix well.
8 Serve with crushed almonds sprinkled on top and season with a pinch of sea salt.

Nutritional Facts:

Calories: 271 | Carbohydrates: 9 g | Protein: 7.57 g | Fat: 1.86 g | Sodium: 182 mg

5.16. Cucumber Soup

Ready In:

- Prep: 10 Min.
- Serving: 2

What you need:

- 1 tbsp garlic
- 1/2 tbsp lemon juice
- 2 cups English cucumbers (peeled and diced, with 1/4 cup reserved for garnish)
- 1/4 cup onions (diced)
- 1 cup vegetable broth
- 1/8 tsp red pepper flakes
- 1/8 cup parsley (diced)
- A pinch of salt
- 1/4 cup Greek yogurt (plain)

Instructions:

1 In a blender, combine garlic, lemon juice, 2 cups diced cucumber, onions, vegetable broth, red pepper flakes, parsley, salt, and Greek yogurt.
2 Blend until completely smooth.
3 Pour the soup into serving bowls.
4 Garnish with the reserved sliced cucumbers and serve chilled.

Nutritional Facts:

Calories: 55 | Carbohydrates: 8.77 g | Protein: 2.33 g | Fat: 1.26 g | Sodium: 436 mg

5.17. Eggplant Salad

Ready In:

- Prep: 8 Min.| Cook: 20 Min.
- Serving: 3

What you need:

- 2 sliced eggplants
- 1/2 cup parsley (chopped)
- 2 cloves of garlic
- 1/2 cup eggless mayonnaise
- 2 green peppers (cut and seeded)
- Salt and black pepper

Instructions:

1. Preheat the oven to 480°F (250°C).
2. Place the sliced eggplants and bell peppers on a baking sheet.
3. Bake for 10 minutes, flipping halfway through the cooking time.
4. In a large mixing bowl, combine the baked eggplants, bell peppers, minced garlic, mayonnaise, and chopped parsley.
5. Mix well, and season with salt and black pepper.
6. Serve chilled or at room temperature.

Nutritional Facts:

Calories: 196 | Carbohydrates: 13.4 g | Protein: 14.6 g | Fat: 10.8 g | Sodium: 156 mg

5.18. Cauliflower, Broccoli, and Carrot Bake

Ready In:

- Prep: 10 Min|Cook: 30 Min.
- Serving: 10

What you need:

- 1 cup carrots
- 1 cup frozen whole small onions or 3 medium onions, quartered
- tbsp olive oil or avocado oil
- cups broccoli (raw)
- 2 tbsp flour (consider whole grain or almond flour for a healthier twist)
- 1 cup almond milk or another non-dairy milk alternative
- 1 package (3 oz) cashew-based cream cheese or another non-dairy alternative, softened
- Dash of pepper
- 2 cups cauliflower (raw)
- 1/2 cup high-quality, organic cheddar cheese, shredded (optional, and ensure moderation)
- 1/2 cup soft whole grain breadcrumbs

Instructions:

1. Wash and slice the vegetables, then steam them until crisp-tender. Drain.
2. In a skillet, heat 2 tablespoons of olive or avocado oil. Stir in flour and pepper.
3. Gradually add almond milk, stirring continuously until the mixture thickens and starts to bubble.
4. Lower the heat and mix in the cashew-based cream cheese until smooth.
5. In a 1.5-quart casserole dish, layer the steamed vegetables. Pour the sauce over and mix gently.
6. Sprinkle the (optional) cheddar cheese on top.
7. Preheat the oven to 350°F and bake for 15 minutes.
8. Mix the whole grain breadcrumbs with the remaining oil and sprinkle over the casserole. Bake for another 15 minutes.

Nutritional Facts: Calories: 120-Carbohydrates: 8 g-Protein: 4 g-Fat: 9 g-Sodium: 90 mg

5.19. Broccoli Blossom

Ready In:

- Prep: 10 Min.| Cook: 10 Min.
- Yields: 4

What you need:

- 1/2 cup onion
- 2 cup chopped red cabbage
- 1 cup chopped broccoli
- 2-3 tbsp water
- 2 tbsp olive oil
- 1/2 tsp garlic powder
- 1/2 tsp onion powder
- Pepper, to taste(black and red)
- 2 whole grain or gluten-free English muffin, split and toasted
- tbsp grated organic Parmesan cheese (use sparingly)

Instructions:

1. In a large pan or wok, heat the olive oil and stir-fry the vegetables for 2-3 minutes.
2. Add water, cover, and let it steam for 5 minutes.
3. In the last 2 minutes, stir in garlic powder, onion powder, and peppers.
4. Serve with toasted whole grain or gluten-free English muffin halves, sparingly sprinkled with Parmesan cheese.

Nutritional Facts: Calories: 180|Carbohydrates: 19 g|Protein: 7 g|Fat: 9 g|Sodium: 110 mg

5.20. Hot German Cabbage

Ready In:

- Prep: 10 Min.| Cook: 15 Min.
- Serving: 4

What you need:

- 2 tbsp honey (instead of sugar for a natural sweetener)
- 1/2 tsp caraway seed
- 1/4 tsp pepper
- 1 tbsp minced onion
- tbsp apple cider vinegar (which can be more beneficial than regular vinegar)
- 1/2 tsp dry mustard
- 2 tbsp olive oil (instead of margarine)
- cups shredded red cabbage
- 1 cup diced green apple (unpeeled)
- The other instructions remain the same.

Instructions

1 Place all Ingredients, except lemon juice, in a 12-inch heavy skillet with a tight-fitting cover.
2 Cook, covered, over medium heat for 15 minutes or until tender-crisp, shaking the pan regularly to avoid sticking.
3 Toss with a squeeze of lemon juice.

Nutritional Facts

Calories: 47| Carbohydrates: 6 g| Protein: 1.5 g| Fat: 2 g| Sodium 228 mg

5.21. Steamed Green Beans

Ready In:

- Prep.: 10 Min| Cook: 15 Min.
- Serving: 4

What you need:

- 1/2 cup diced sweet red pepper
- 1/2 tsp basil
- 1 tbsp vegetable oil
- 2 tbsp water
- 1 lb green beans, trimmed
- 1/4 tsp pepper
- 1 tbsp lemon juice

Instructions

1 Combine all ingredients, except the lemon juice, in a 12-inch heavy skillet with a tight-fitting lid.
2 Cook, covered, over medium heat for 15 minutes or until beans are tender-crisp. Shake the skillet occasionally to prevent sticking.
3 Before serving, toss with lemon juice.

Nutritional Facts

Calories: 48 | Carbohydrates: 7 g | Protein: 2 g | Fat: 1.8 g | Sodium: 228 mg

Chapter 6: Fish Recipes

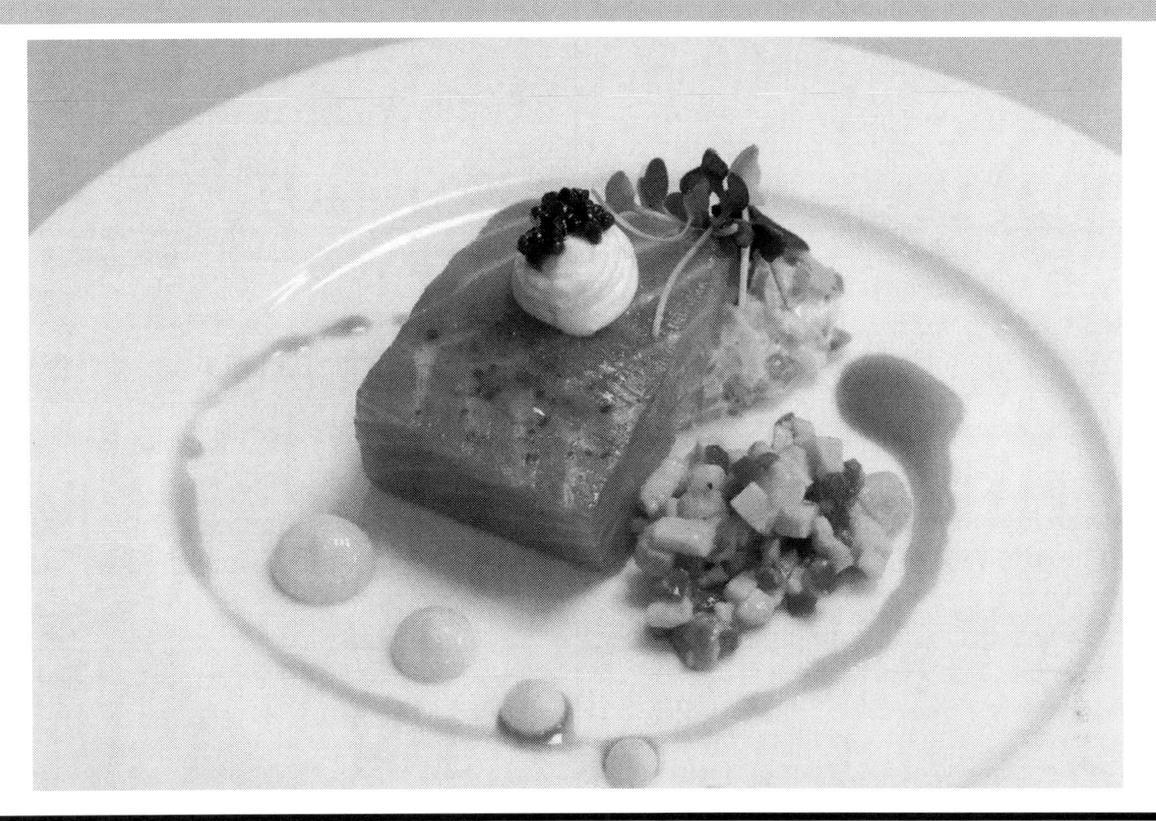

6.1. Juicy Salmon Dish

Ready In:

- Prep: 6 Min. | Cook: 15 Min.
- Yields: For One

What you need:

- 1/4 cup water
- Few sprigs of parsley, basil, and tarragon
- 0.5 pounds salmon (skin on)
- 1 tsp of olive oil
- 1 tsp salt
- 2 tbsp pepper
- 1/4 lemon (thinly sliced)
- 0.5 whole carrot (julienned)

Instructions

1. In a saucepan, add water and herbs, then bring to a simmer.
2. In a separate pan, heat olive oil over medium heat. Season salmon with salt and pepper, then place it skin-side down in the pan. Place slices of lemon on top.
3. Cook salmon for 3-4 minutes on each side, or until it's cooked through but still moist inside.
4. In the saucepan with herbs, add julienned carrots. Sauté for 1-2 minutes until slightly tender.
5. Serve salmon with sautéed carrots and garnish with additional herbs if desired.

Nutritional Values:

Calories: 455 | Carbohydrates: 3 g | Protein: 34 g | Fat: 33 g | Sodium: 150 mg

6.2. Fish with Peppers

Ready In:

- Prep: 10 Min. | Cook: 25 Min.
- Serving: 5

What you need:

- 1 1/2 lb. fish fillets
- 1 tsp garlic powder
- 1/2 cup low-sodium chicken broth
- 1/4 cup no-salt-added tomato sauce
- 1 tsp capers
- 2 tbsp oil
- 1/2 tsp lemon pepper
- 1/2 medium green pepper (cut into rings)
- 1/2 medium red pepper (cut into rings)

Instructions

1. Cut the fish into 4-inch chunks.
2. In a large pan, heat the oil over medium heat. Add fish and cook for about 5 minutes on each side or until browned.
3. Add garlic powder, chicken broth, tomato sauce, capers, and lemon pepper to the pan.
4. Place pepper rings on top of the fish.
5. Cover the pan and simmer for about 15 minutes or until the fish flakes easily with a fork and the peppers are tender.

Nutritional Facts

Calories: 207 | Carbohydrates: 9 g | Protein: 25 g | Fat: 12 g | Sodium: 136 mg

6.3. Herb Topped Fish

Ready In:

- Prep: 8 Min.| Cook: 20 Min.
- Serving: 6

What you need:

- 1-1/2-inch-thick pieces of salmon, halibut or other white fish (24 oz.)
- 1/2 cup avocado-based mayo
- 1/4 cup grated Parmesan cheese
- tbsp chives (chopped)
- 1/2 cup sour cream
- 2 tbsp parsley (chopped)
- 1/2 tsp onion powder
- 1/2 tsp dry mustard
- Fresh ground pepper to taste
- 1/2 tsp dried dill

Instructions

1. Preheat the oven to 350°F.
2. Place uncooked fish fillets in a greased shallow baking pan.
3. In a mixing bowl, combine avocado mayo, Parmesan, chives, sour cream, parsley, onion powder, dry mustard, pepper, and dill.
4. Spread the mixture evenly over the tops of the fish fillets.
5. Bake for 20 minutes or until the fish flakes easily with a fork.

Nutritional Values:

Calories: 240 | Carbohydrates: 2 g | Protein: 20g | Fat: 15 g | Sodium: 126 mg

6.4. Fish Cakes

Ready In:

- Prep: 12min. | Cook: 15 Min.
- Serving: 6

What you need:

- 1 lb. haddock (cooked and flaked)
- 1-2 tsp lemon juice
- 1/2 cup plain bread crumbs
- 2 eggs (beaten)
- 3 cups mashed potatoes
- Paprika and pepper to flavor

Instructions

1. Set the oven temperature to 375°F.
2. Toss flaked haddock with lemon juice.
3. In a mixing bowl, combine the haddock with mashed potatoes, pepper, and paprika.
4. Form into 6 cakes, about 1 inch thick.
5. Dip each cake into the beaten egg, then roll in breadcrumbs.
6. Place on a cookie sheet and bake for 15 minutes or until golden brown and cooked through.

Nutritional Facts

Calories: 152 | Carbohydrates: 16 g | Protein: 20 g | Fat: 22 g | Sodium: 186 mg

6.5. Salmon Pasta with Butter

Ready In:

- Prep: 7 Min. | Cook: 15 Min.
- Serving: 4

What you need:

- 350g Salmon fillets
- 600ml Water
- 400g Dried pasta
- 15g Butter
- 2 tbsp Plain flour
- 2 tbsp fresh tarragon (chopped)
- 1 Bay leaf
- Black pepper to taste

Instructions

1. In a saucepan, poach the salmon fillets with the bay leaf in water for about 15 minutes or until fully cooked. Once done, remove the fish and reserve 450ml of the cooking liquid.
2. While the salmon is poaching, boil the pasta in a large pot until al dente.
3. Flake the poached salmon, discarding the skin and any bones.
4. In a separate small saucepan, melt the butter, then whisk in the flour. Cook for about a minute.
5. Gradually stir in the reserved fish cooking liquid. Return to heat, whisking continuously until the sauce thickens.
6. Season with black pepper and stir in the chopped tarragon.
7. Drain the pasta, combine it with the salmon and sauce, and toss gently until well-mixed.

Nutritional Facts

Calories: 394| Carbohydrates: 30 g| Protein: 27 g| Fat: 15 g| Sodium 126 mg

6.6. Salmon with Pineapple Salsa

Ready In:

- ➢ Prep: 10 Min. | Cook: 20 Min.
- ➢ Serving: 6

What you need:

- 1 1/2 pounds salmon fillets
- Marinade:
- 1/2 clove garlic (minced)
- 2 tbsp brown sugar
- 1/4 cup unsweetened pineapple juice
- 1/4 tsp ground ginger
- 2 tbsp low-salt soy sauce
- 1 1/2 tbsp apple cider vinegar
- Pineapple salsa:
- 1/4 cup red pepper (finely chopped)
- 2 tbsp red onion (finely chopped)
- 1 cup fresh pineapple (chopped)
- 2 tbsp fresh cilantro (finely chopped)

Instructions

1. For the marinade, mix together soy sauce, garlic, ginger, brown sugar, pineapple juice, and apple cider vinegar in a bowl.
2. Reserve 2 tbsp of the marinade and place the salmon in the rest. Ensure the fish is well-coated, then refrigerate for at least 15 minutes to marinate.
3. In a separate bowl, combine the reserved marinade with red pepper, red onion, pineapple, and cilantro. Mix well to form the pineapple salsa.
4. Remove the salmon from the refrigerator and discard any excess marinade.
5. Grill the salmon over medium-high heat, about 6-7 minutes on each side or until it easily flakes. Baste with the reserved 2 tbsp of marinade while grilling.
6. Serve grilled salmon with a generous serving of pineapple salsa on the side.

Nutritional Facts: KCal: 185| Carb.: 8 g| Protein: 22 g| Fat: 24 g| Sodium 136 mg

6.7. Smoked Haddock with Lentils

Ready In:

- ➢ Prep: 25 Min. | Cook: 20 Min.
- ➢ Serving: 2

What you need:

- 2 tbsp of olive oil
- ½ medium onion (finely chopped)
- 1 celery stick (finely sliced)
- 1 carrot (diagonally sliced)
- 1 rosemary sprig or ¼ tsp dried rosemary
- 1 garlic clove (finely sliced)
- 250g cooked lentils
- 200ml vegetable stock (made with ½ stock cube)
- 140g smoked haddock or cod fillets (skinned)
- A small handful of parsley leaves (chopped)

Instructions

1. In a non-stick frying pan or saucepan, heat olive oil over low heat. Add the onion, celery, and carrot, and sauté until soft, about 5 minutes.
2. Stir in the rosemary and garlic, cooking briefly.
3. Add the lentils and pour in the vegetable stock. Bring the mixture to a gentle simmer.
4. Place the fish fillets on top of the lentils, cover with a lid, and cook for about 8 minutes or until the fish starts to flake when tested with a knife.
5. Season with freshly ground black pepper, garnish with chopped parsley, and serve.

Nutritional Facts

Calories: 494| Carbohydrates: 0 g| Protein: 16 g| Fat: 21 g| Sodium 29 mg

6.8. Pan-Fried Fish with Lemon and Parsley

Ready In:

- Prep: 30 Min. | Cook: 20 Min.
- Serving: 1

What you need:

- 1 plaice fillet
- 15g butter
- 1 tbsp of olive oil
- 1 tbsp lemon juice
- Small bunch of fresh parsley (chopped)

Instructions

1. Season the plaice fillet with salt and black pepper.
2. In a non-stick frying pan, melt butter and olive oil over medium heat.
3. Place the fillet skin-side down and cook for about 3 minutes. Gently turn and cook the other side for 1-2 minutes or until fully cooked.
4. Transfer the fish to a serving plate.
5. In the same pan, add lemon juice and parsley. Whisk and cook for a few seconds. Pour this buttery mixture over the cooked fish and serve.

Nutritional Facts

Calories: 367| Carbohydrates: 25 g| Protein: 33 g| Fat: 13 g| Sodium 125 mg

6.9. Crunchy Fish Bites

Ready In:

- Prep: 25 Min. | Cook: 20 Min.
- Yields: 2

What you need:

- 1 medium egg
- 40 grams quick-cook polenta (fine cornmeal)
- 20 grams of ground almonds
- 275 grams thick skinless white fish fillet (such as cod, haddock or Pollock), cut into roughly 3cm chunks
- 2 tablespoons olive or rapeseed oil
- Lemon wedges, to serve

Instructions

1. In a small bowl, whisk the egg and season with salt and pepper.
2. In a separate bowl, combine the polenta and almonds. Season with black pepper and sea salt.
3. Coat the fish pieces in the beaten egg, then toss in the polenta mixture. Place on a platter and set aside.
4. Heat a large non-stick frying pan over medium and add the oil.
5. Fry the fish bites for 5–7 minutes or until golden brown, crisp, and cooked through, turning occasionally.
6. Serve with lemon wedges on the side.

Nutritional Facts

Calories: 384| Carbohydrates: 15 g| Protein: 33 g| Fat: 0.5 g| Sodium 99 mg

6.10. Mediterranean Fish Bake

Ready In:

- Prep: 20 Min. | Cook: 25 Min.
- Yields: 2

What you need:

- 1 medium red onion, cut into 12 segments
- 1 red pepper, cut into 2cm chunks
- 1 courgette, halved lengthways and cut into 2cm chunks
- 2 medium tomatoes, quartered
- 1½ tablespoon olive oil
- 100 grams of sea bass or sea bream fillets
- 40 grams pitted black olives (preferably Kalamata), drained
- Juice ½ large lemon, plus extra wedges to serve

Instructions

1. Preheat the oven to 200°C.
2. Scatter the onion, pepper, courgette, and tomato quarters on a large baking tray.
3. Drizzle with 1 tablespoon of oil and season. Roast for 20 minutes.
4. Add the fish skin-side down among the vegetables. Squeeze lemon juice over, then scatter the olives.
5. Return to the oven for about 10 minutes, or until the fish is cooked through.
6. Serve drizzled with the remaining oil and accompanied by lemon wedges.

Nutritional Facts

Calories: 274| Carbohydrates: 22 g| Protein: 11 g| Fat: 26 g| Sodium 146 mg

6.11. Ginger and Chili Baked Fish

Ready In:

- Prep: 30 Min.| Cook: 20 Min.
- Serving: 1

What you need:

- 175 grams thick white fish fillet
- 1 garlic clove, thinly sliced
- 15 grams of stem ginger
- 1 spring onion
- 2 teaspoon of olive oil
- 1 red bird's eye chili
- ½ small lime
- Fresh coriander leaves, to garnish

Instructions

1. Preheat the oven to 200°C.
2. Place the fish on a baking tray lined with foil, ensuring there's enough foil to enclose it.
3. Top the fish with garlic, ginger, spring onion, and chili. Squeeze lime juice over.
4. Season, then fold the foil over the fish, sealing the edges to form a pouch.
5. Bake for about 20 minutes or until the fish is cooked through.
6. Serve with fresh coriander and lime wedges.

Nutritional Facts

Calories: 233| Carbohydrates: 7 g| Protein: 31 g| Fat: 11 g| Sodium 346 mg

6.12. Crusted Whitefish

Ready In:

- Prep:8 Minutes | Cook: 20 Min.
- Yields: 4

What you need:

- Half a cup of pistachios
- 2 tablespoons of parsley
- 2 tablespoons of cheese
- 2 tablespoons of breadcrumbs
- 4 tablespoons of olive oil
- Half teaspoon of salt
- 40 ounces of skinless white fish

Instructions

1. Preheat the oven to 350°F and position the center rack.
2. Line a baking sheet with foil.
3. Blend all ingredients except fish in a food processor until nuts are finely crushed.
4. Place fish on the baking sheet and evenly spread the nut mixture over it, pressing down gently.
5. Bake for 20-30 minutes or until the fish flakes easily with a fork. Adjust baking time based on the thickness of the fish fillet.

Nutritional Facts

Calories: 275| Carbohydrates: 4 g| Protein: 20 g| Fat: 20 g| Sodium 186 mg

6.13. Turmeric-Infused Shellfish in Wine

Ready In:

- Prep: 8 Min.| Cook: 20 Min.
- Yields: 2

What you need:

- 2-lbs fresh cuttlefish
- ½-cup extra-virgin olive oil
- 1 large onion, finely chopped
- 1-cup Roble white wine
- ¼-cup lukewarm water
- 1 bay leaf
- ½-bunch fresh cilantro , chopped
- 4 tomatoes, grated
- 1 tsp turmeric powder
- Salt (preferably pink Himalayan) and pepper to taste
- 1 tbsp freshly grated ginger

Instructions:

1. Start by cleaning the cuttlefish: Remove its hard cartilage centerpiece (cuttlebone), ink bag, and guts. Then, wash the cuttlefish under running water.
2. Slice the cleaned cuttlefish into thin pieces and drain any excess water.
3. In a saucepan on medium-high heat, warm the oil and sauté the onion and grated ginger until aromatic, roughly 3 minutes.
4. Add the cuttlefish slices to the pan and pour in the white wine. Allow it to simmer for 5 minutes.
5. Incorporate the lukewarm water, grated tomatoes, bay leaf, turmeric powder, chopped cilantro, salt, and pepper. Occasionally stir and allow cooking until the cuttlefish becomes tender and the sauce has thickened.
6. As with the original recipe, be cautious not to overcook the cuttlefish to maintain its delicate texture. If desired, briefly grill the cuttlefish for 3 minutes over a fire before incorporating it into the dish.
7. Serve warm, preferably with brown rice or quinoa (both known for their health benefits).

Nutritional Facts:

Calories: 235 | Carbohydrates: 9 g | Protein: 13 g | Fat: 18 g | Sodium: 200 mg

6.14. Pistachio Fish

Ready In:

- ➢ Prep: 5 Min.| Cook: 10 Min.
- ➢ Yields: 2

What you need:

- 4 (5 ounces) boneless sole fillets
- ½ cup pistachios, finely chopped
- Juice of 1 lemon
- 1 teaspoon extra virgin olive oil
- Salt and pepper for seasoning

Instructions:

1. Preheat the oven to a suitable temperature for fish baking, ideally 375°F (190°C).
2. Line a baking sheet with parchment paper.
3. Pat the sole fillets dry with kitchen towels and season them with salt and pepper.
4. In a separate bowl, prepare your pistachios.
5. Lay the fillets on the baking sheet and sprinkle each with the chopped pistachios. Drizzle the lemon juice and olive oil over the top.
6. Bake in the preheated oven for about 10 minutes, or until the fillets turn golden brown and flake easily when tested with a fork.

Nutritional Facts:

Calories: 143.7 | Carbohydrates: 34.62 g | Protein: 3.44 g | Fat: 3.19 g | Sodium: 236 mg

6.15. Herb-Crusted Tilapia

Ready In:

- ➢ Prep: 10 Min.| Cook: 15 Min
- ➢ Yields: 2

What you need:

- 2 (6 ounces) tilapia fillets
- 1 tablespoon extra-virgin olive oil
- ½ cup almond flour
- 1 tablespoon fresh parsley, finely chopped
- 1 teaspoon dried oregano
- 1 garlic clove, minced
- Zest of 1 lemon
- Salt and pepper to taste

Instructions:

1. Preheat your oven to 400°F (205°C).
2. Brush both sides of the tilapia fillets with olive oil.
3. In a mixing bowl, combine almond flour, parsley, oregano, garlic, lemon zest, salt, and pepper.
4. Dredge each tilapia fillet in the herb mixture, ensuring it's well-coated.
5. Place the fillets on a parchment-lined baking tray.
6. Bake for 12-15 minutes, or until the fish flakes easily with a fork.
7. Serve hot with a wedge of lemon and steamed vegetables.

Nutritional Facts:

Calories: 285 | Carbohydrates: 6 g | Protein: 34 g | Fat: 13 g | Sodium: 150 mg

6.16. Grilled Mahi Mahi with Mango Salsa

Ready In:

- Prep: 20 Min.| Cook: 10 Min.
- Yields: 2

What you need:

- 2 (6 ounces) mahi mahi fillets
- 1 tablespoon avocado oil
- 1 ripe mango, diced
- ¼ cup red bell pepper, finely chopped
- ¼ cup red onion, finely chopped
- 1 tablespoon fresh cilantro, chopped
- Juice of 1 lime
- Salt and pepper to taste

Instructions:

1. Preheat your grill to medium-high heat.
2. Brush the mahi mahi fillets with avocado oil and season with salt and pepper.
3. Grill the fillets for about 4-5 minutes on each side, or until fully cooked.
4. For the salsa, mix together mango, red bell pepper, red onion, cilantro, lime juice, salt, and pepper in a bowl.
5. Serve the grilled mahi mahi hot with a generous topping of mango salsa.

Nutritional Facts:

Calories: 310 | Carbohydrates: 23 g | Protein: 34 g | Fat: 10 g | Sodium: 130 mg

6.17. Cod in Ginger and Turmeric Broth

Ready In:

- Prep: 8 Min. | Cook: 20 Min.
- Yields: 2

What you need:

- 2 (6 ounces) cod fillets
- 2 cups bone broth or vegetable broth
- 1-inch ginger, thinly sliced
- 1 teaspoon ground turmeric
- 1 tablespoon coconut oil
- 1 small red chili, finely chopped (optional)
- 2 green onions, thinly sliced
- Salt to taste

Instructions:

1. In a pot, heat the coconut oil over medium heat. Add ginger slices and sauté for 2 minutes.
2. Add the bone broth, ground turmeric, and salt. Bring the mixture to a boil.
3. Once boiling, reduce the heat to a simmer, and place the cod fillets into the pot.
4. Let the fish cook for 10-12 minutes or until it's cooked through and flakes easily.
5. Serve the cod in bowls, ladled with the aromatic broth. Garnish with red chili and green onions.

Nutritional Facts:

Calories: 270 | Carbohydrates: 5 g | Protein: 34 g | Fat: 12 g | Sodium: 700 mg

Chapter 7: Snacks Recipes

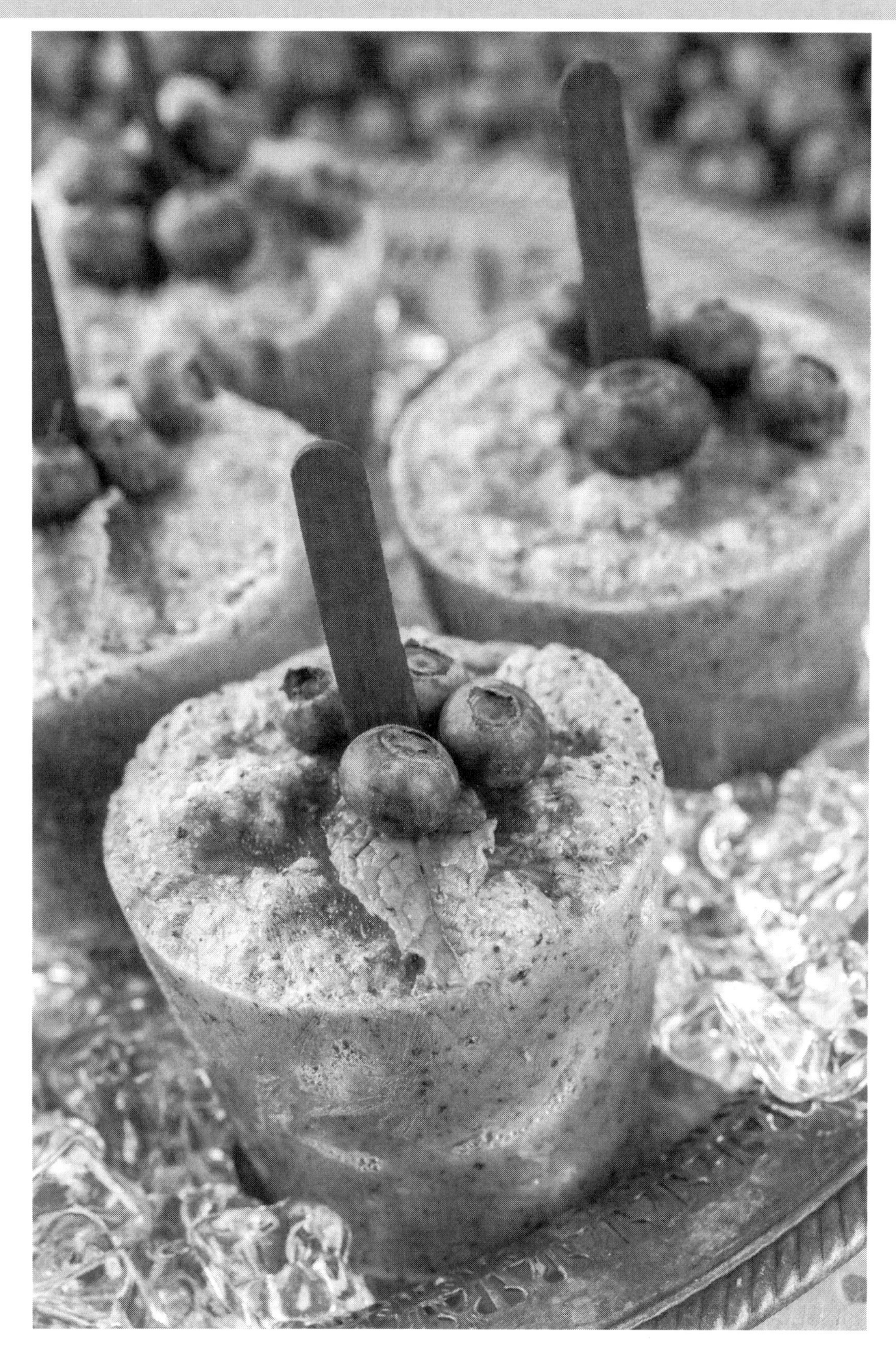

7.1. Blueberries and Cream Ice Pops

Ready in:

- Preparation time: 10 minutes + 3 hours to freeze
- Serving: 6

What you need:

- cups fresh blueberries
- 1 tsp freshly squeezed lemon juice
- ¼ cup unsweetened rice milk
- ¼ cup granulated sugar
- ½ tsp pure vanilla extract
- ¼ cup light sour cream
- ¼ tsp ground cinnamon

Instructions:

1. Puree the blueberries, lemon juice, rice milk, sour cream, sugar, vanilla, and cinnamon in a blender until smooth.
2. Pour the mixture into ice pop molds, filling each mold halfway. Freeze for 3 to 4 hours, or until completely solidified.

Nutritional Facts:

Calories 78 | Carbohydrates 18g | Protein 1g | Fat 1g | Sodium 12 mg

7.2. Candied Ginger Ice Milk

Ready in:

- Prep.: 20 minutes + 1 hour to infuse + 1 hour to freeze
- Cook: 20 minutes
- Serving: 4

What you need:

- cups vanilla rice milk
- ½ cup granulated sugar
- ¼ tsp ground nutmeg
- 1 (4-inch) piece of fresh ginger (peeled and sliced thin)
- ¼ cup finely chopped candied ginger

Instructions:

1. In a large saucepan over medium heat, combine the rice milk, sugar, and fresh ginger slices. Heat the mixture for about 5 minutes, or until nearly boiling, stirring constantly.
2. Reduce heat to low and simmer for 15 minutes. Remove from heat and stir in the nutmeg. Allow the mixture to infuse for 1 hour. Strain the milk mixture through a fine strainer to discard the ginger slices.
3. Cool the mixture in the refrigerator. Once cooled, add the chopped candied ginger. Use an ice cream maker to churn the mixture according to the manufacturer's instructions.
4. Store the ice milk in an airtight container and freeze for up to 3 months.

Nutritional Facts:

Calories 108 | Carbohydrates 24g | Protein 0g | Fat 1g | Sodium 47 mg

7.3. Strawberry-Mango Parfaits with Ginger Topping

Ready in:

- Prep: 5 minutes
- Serving: 4

What you need:

- 1-pint fresh strawberries (stemmed and sliced)
- tbsp granulated sugar
- ½ cup gingersnap crumbs
- 1 pint light or reduced-fat strawberry ice cream
- 2 tbsp orange juice
- 1 pint mango/orange sorbet
- 2 tsp orange rind (grated)
- 2 tbsp crystallized ginger (coarsely chopped, optional)

Instructions:

1. Combine strawberries, sugar, juice, and orange rind in a bowl. In 4 deep

bowls or parfait glasses, alternate layers of sorbet and ice cream.
2 Drizzle the strawberry sauce over each layer.
3 Top with gingersnap crumbs and, if desired, the chopped crystallized ginger.

Nutritional Facts:

Calories 380 | Carbohydrates 78g | Proteins 4g | Fats 7.2g | Sodium 142 mg

7.4. Chocolate Chip Cookies

Ready In:

- Prep: 8 Min.
- Cook: 18-20 Min.
- Serving: 6

What you need:

- 1 cup blanched almond flour (sifted)
- 3 tbsp melted coconut oil
- 1/8 tsp baking soda
- 1/4 tsp cinnamon
- 2 tbsp honey
- 1 1/2 tsp vanilla
- ¼ tsp or less sea salt (to taste)
- ¼ cup Enjoy Life Chocolate Chips or chopped dark chocolate (70-85 percent or higher)

Instructions:

1. Preheat the oven to 350°F. In a mixing bowl, combine almond flour, sea salt, baking soda, and cinnamon.
2. In another bowl, mix together the coconut oil, honey, and vanilla. Slowly pour the wet ingredients into the dry ones, mixing until well combined.
3. Fold in the chocolate chips. Drop by spoonful onto a baking sheet and flatten slightly. Bake for 10-11 minutes, or until edges are golden brown.

Nutritional Facts:

Calories 230 | Carbohydrates 13g | Proteins 5g | Fats 19.1g | Sodium 128 mg

7.5. Strawberry Lime Dessert

Ready in:

- Prep: 10 minutes
- Cook: 0 minutes (No cooking needed)
- Serving: 6

What you need:

- cups fresh strawberries (stems removed and quartered)
- 1/2 cup whipping cream
- 1 tablespoon sugar
- 1/4 teaspoon lime peel zest
- 1 lime (cut into 6-8 wedges)

Instructions

1 In a shallow dish, mash 1 cup of the quartered strawberries using a potato masher or puree using a blender.
2 In a medium mixing bowl, whip the cream, sugar, and lime peel together until stiff peaks form.
3 Layer the whipped cream mixture and the remaining strawberries in 6 separate 6- to 7-ounce cups or glasses.
4 Serve each with a slice of fresh lime on top.
5 Enjoy immediately or refrigerate for up to 2 hours before serving.

Nutritional Facts

Calories 90 | Carbohydrates 9 g | Proteins 1 g | Fats 6.4 g | Sodium 8 mg |

7.6. Light and Creamy Cranberry Fresh Fruit Dip

Ready in:

- Prep: 5 minutes
- Cook: 0 minutes (No cooking needed)
- Serving: 12

What you need:

- ounces light sour cream
- 1/2 cup whole-berry cranberry sauce
- 1/4 teaspoon nutmeg
- 1/4 teaspoon ground ginger

Instructions

1 Combine all ingredients in a blender or food processor.
2 Blend until smooth.
3 Serve with fresh fruits like pineapple, pears, or strawberries.

Nutritional Facts

Calories 45 | Carbohydrates 7 g | Proteins 1 g | Fats 1.2 g | Sodium 21 mg |

7.7. Blackberry Cobbler

Ready in:

- Prep: 5 minutes
- Cook: 30-35 minutes
- Serving: 6

What you need:

- Vegetable oil cooking spray
- 1/2 cup all-purpose flour
- 1 12-ounce bag frozen unsweetened blackberries, thawed
- 1/4 cup granulated sugar
- 1 1/2 tablespoons cornstarch
- 1 1/2 tablespoons water
- 3/4 cup quick oats
- 1/2 teaspoon ground cinnamon
- 1/2 cup unsalted butter, softened
- 2/3 cup firmly packed brown sugar
- 1 8-ounce container light or reduced-fat whipped cream

Instructions

1 Preheat the oven to 350°F. Lightly spray an 8-inch square baking dish with cooking spray.
2 In a large pot, combine the blackberries and sugar and let sit for 30 minutes.
3 Cook the blackberry-sugar mixture over medium heat, stirring occasionally, for 5 minutes.
4 In a separate bowl, mix the water and cornstarch until smooth. Add this mixture to the blackberries.
5 Bring to a boil over medium-high heat, then reduce to a simmer for 1 minute or until the mixture thickens.
6 Transfer the mixture to the prepared baking dish.
7 In another bowl, combine the flour, oats, cinnamon, softened butter, and brown sugar. Mix until crumbly.
8 Evenly spread this mixture over the blackberry layer.
9 Bake for 25-30 minutes or until golden brown and bubbly.
10 Serve warm, topped with whipped cream.

Nutritional Facts

Calories 320 | Carbohydrates 48 g | Proteins 3 g | Fats 13.6 g | Sodium 8 mg |

7.8. Coconut Angel Food Cake

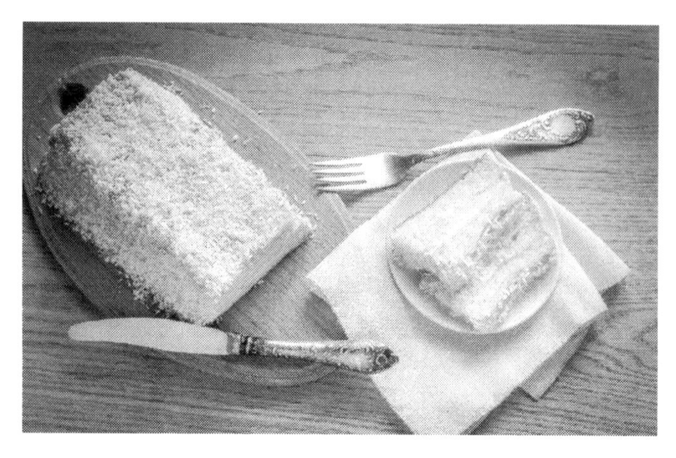

Ready In:

- Prep: 12 Min.
- Cook: 22 Min.
- Serving: 12
-

What you need:

Cake:

- 1 1/4 cups egg whites
- 1 teaspoon cream of tartar
- 1 cup superfine sugar
- teaspoons pure vanilla extract
- 1/3 cup dried, unsweetened coconut shavings
- 1/4 teaspoon salt
- teaspoons fresh lemon juice
- 1 cup sifted cake flour

Sauce:

- 1 bag cranberries
- 2/3 cup granulated sugar
- 2/3 cup fresh orange juice
- tablespoons orange-flavored liqueur
- 1 tablespoon grated orange zest
- ½ teaspoon cinnamon

Instructions

Cake:

1. Preheat the oven to 325°F.
2. In a large mixing bowl, beat the egg whites and salt until frothy. Add cream of tartar and continue beating until soft peaks form.
3. Gradually add 1/2 cup of sugar, one tablespoon at a time, beating until soft glossy peaks form.
4. Gently fold in vanilla and lemon juice.
5. In a separate bowl, combine the remaining sugar and flour. Gently fold this mixture into the egg whites, then fold in the dried coconut.
6. Transfer the batter into a 10-inch ungreased angel food tube pan.
7. Bake for 20-22 minutes or until the top is lightly browned and springs back when touched.
8. Invert the pan onto the neck of a bottle to cool. Once cooled, run a knife around the pan to release the cake.

Sauce:

1. In a medium saucepan, combine all the sauce ingredients and bring to a boil.
2. Reduce heat and simmer until slightly thickened.
3. Cool the sauce, then refrigerate for at least 1 hour.
4. Serve the cake slices with 3 tablespoons of the sauce and sprinkle with extra coconut shavings.

Nutritional Facts

Calories 215 | Carbohydrates 44 g | Proteins 4 g | Fats 2.4 g | Sodium 94 mg |

7.9 Lemon Ricotta Pie

Ready in:

- Prep: 15 mins - Cooking: 25 mins
- Serving: 8

What you need:

- large eggs (separated)
- Juice and zest of 1 medium lemon
- 15 oz ricotta cheese (part-skim; whole can be used as well)
- 2/3 cup natural sweetener (like stevia or monk fruit extract)
- 1/2 tsp vanilla
- Dash of salt

Instructions:

1. Preheat the oven to 350°F.
2. In a separate bowl, whisk egg whites until soft peaks form.
3. In another bowl, combine egg yolks, ricotta, lemon juice, lemon zest, sweetener, vanilla, and salt.
4. Taste the mixture. If you want a stronger lemon flavor, feel free to add a bit more zest or juice.
5. Gently fold the egg whites into the ricotta mixture.
6. Pour the blend into a prepared pie pan.
7. Bake for 25 minutes. Test with a wooden skewer – it should come out clean.
8. Let it cool completely before slicing into 8 pieces. Best served with fresh berries or your favorite topping.

Nutritional Values:

Calories: 105 | Carbohydrates: 4g | Proteins: 8g | Fats: 6.2g | Sodium: 127mg

7.10. Meringue Cookies

Ready in:

- Prep: 30 mins - Cook: 30 mins
- Serving: 24

What you need:

- egg whites (room temperature)
- 1 cup granulated sugar
- 1 tsp pure vanilla extract
- 1 tsp almond extract

Instructions:

1. Preheat the oven to 300°F. Prepare 2 baking sheets lined with parchment paper.
2. In a large stainless-steel bowl, whisk egg whites until they form firm peaks.
3. Gradually add sugar, 1 tablespoon at a time, whisking well after each addition, until the meringue is thick and glossy.
4. Gently fold in vanilla and almond extracts.
5. Using a tablespoon, drop the meringue onto the baking sheets, spacing them evenly. Bake for approximately 30 minutes, or until cookies are crisp.
6. Remove from the oven and cool on wire racks. Store in an airtight container at room temperature for up to a week.

Nutritional Values:

Calories: 36 | Carbohydrates: 8g | Protein: 1g | Fat: 0g | Sodium: 9mg

7.11. Corn Bread

Ready in:

- Prep: 10 mins - Cook: 20 mins
- Serving: 10

What you need:

- Cooking spray
- ¾ cup all-purpose flour
- 1 tbsp baking soda
- 1¼ cup yellow cornmeal
- ½ cup granulated sugar
- eggs
- 1 cup unsweetened rice milk (unfortified)
- 2 tbsp olive oil

Instructions:

1. Preheat the oven to 425°F. Prepare an 8-by-8-inch baking dish with a light spray of cooking spray.
2. In a medium bowl, mix cornmeal, flour, baking soda, and sugar.
3. In a separate bowl, whisk together eggs, rice milk, and olive oil.
4. Combine wet and dry ingredients and whisk until smooth.
5. Pour batter into the baking dish and bake for 20 minutes, or until it turns golden.
6. Best served warm.

Nutritional Values:

Calories: 198 | Carbohydrates: 34g | Protein: 4g | Fat: 5g | Sodium: 25mg

7.12. Roasted Red Pepper and Chicken Crostini

Ready in:

- Prep: 10 mins - Cooking: 5 mins
- Serving: 4
-

What you need:

- tbsp olive oil
- slices of French bread
- ½ tsp minced garlic
- 1 roasted red bell pepper (chopped)
- oz cooked chicken breast (shredded)
- ½ cup fresh basil (chopped)

Instructions:

1. Preheat the oven to 400°F. Line a baking pan with aluminum foil.
2. Mix olive oil and garlic in a small bowl.
3. Brush both sides of each bread slice with the olive oil mixture.
4. Lay bread slices on the baking pan and toast for about 5 minutes, turning once, until both sides are golden and crispy.
5. In a medium bowl, mix red pepper, chicken, and basil.
6. Top each toasted bread slice with the red pepper and chicken mixture.

Nutritional Values:

Calories: 184 | Carbohydrates: 19g | Protein: 9g | Fat: 8g | Sodium: 175mg

7.13. Cucumber Wrapped Vegetable Rolls

Ready in:

- Prep: 30 minutes
- Serving: 8

What you need:

- ½ cup finely shredded red cabbage
- ½ cup grated carrot
- ¼ cup chopped cilantro
- ¼ cup julienned scallion (both green and white parts)
- ¼ cup julienned red bell pepper
- 1 tbsp olive oil
- ¼ tsp ground cumin
- ¼ tsp freshly ground black pepper
- 1 English cucumber (sliced into 8 very thin strips with a vegetable peeler)

Instructions:

1. Toss the cabbage, carrot, red pepper, scallion, cilantro, olive oil, cumin, and black pepper in a medium mixing bowl until thoroughly combined.
2. Place an even amount of the vegetable filling at one end of each cucumber strip. Roll up the cucumber strips securing with a wooden pick. Repeat with all cucumber strips.

Nutritional Facts:

Calories 26 | Carbohydrates 3g | Protein 0g | Fat 2g | Sodium 7 mg

7.14. Antojitos

Ready In:

- Prep: 20 Min.
- Cook: 1 H
- Serving: 8

What you need:

- oz plain cream cheese (at room temperature)
- ½ jalapeño pepper (finely chopped)
- ½ tsp ground cumin
- ½ scallion, green part only (chopped)
- ¼ cup finely chopped red bell pepper
- ½ tsp ground coriander
- ½ tsp chili powder
- (8-inch) flour tortillas

Instructions:

1. In a medium mixing bowl, combine the cream cheese, jalapeño pepper, scallion, red bell pepper, cumin, coriander, and chili powder.
2. Spread an equal amount of the cream cheese mixture onto each of the three tortillas, leaving a ¼-inch border around the edges.
3. Roll each tortilla tightly, then wrap securely in plastic wrap. Chill for approximately 1 hour or until firm. Slice each tortilla roll into 1-inch pieces to serve.

Nutritional Facts:

Calories 110 | Carbohydrates 7g | Protein 2g | Fat 8g | Sodium 215 mg

7.15. Cocoa Fat Bombs

Ready in:

- Prep: 10 minutes
- Cook: 5 minutes
- Serving: 8

What you need:

- 1/4 cup cocoa butter
- 1/4 cup coconut oil
- 1/2 tsp vanilla
- drops of liquid Stevia

Instructions:

1. In a small saucepan, melt the cocoa butter and coconut oil over low heat. Once melted, remove from heat and stir in vanilla and Stevia.
2. Pour the mixture into silicone molds and refrigerate until set. Once firm, remove from molds and serve.

Nutritional Facts:
Calories 120 | Carbohydrates 0 g | Protein 0 g | Fat 13.6 g | Sodium 105 mg

7.16. Almond Peanut Butter Bars

Ready in:

- Prep: 10 min.-Cook: 30 min.
- Serving: 10

What you need:

- eggs
- 1/2 cup Swerve
- 1/2 cup butter (softened)
- 1/2 cup peanut butter
- 1 tbsp coconut flour
- 1/4 cup almond flour
- 1/2 tsp vanilla

Instructions:

1. Preheat the oven to 350°F. In a mixing bowl, whisk together eggs, butter, and peanut butter until smooth. Fold in Swerve, coconut flour, almond flour, and vanilla.
2. Pour the mixture into a greased baking pan and smooth the surface. Bake for 30 minutes or until golden brown. Once cooled, cut into bars and serve.

Nutritional Facts:
Calories 190 | Carbohydrates 3.9 g | Protein 5.1 g | Fat 18 g | Sodium 75 mg

7.17. Healthy Protein Bars

Ready in:

- Prep: 10 minutes
- Chill time: 30 minutes
- Serving: 10

What you need:

- scoops of vanilla protein powder
- 1/4 cup melted coconut oil
- 1 cup almond butter
- 1 tsp cinnamon
- 18 drops of liquid Stevia
- Pinch of salt

Instructions:

1. In a mixing bowl, combine the vanilla protein powder, melted coconut oil, almond butter, cinnamon, liquid Stevia, and a pinch of salt.
2. Mix all the ingredients until they come together in a smooth, consistent mixture.
3. Transfer the mixture to a greased or parchment paper-lined baking pan, spreading it out evenly.
4. Place the pan in the refrigerator and allow the mixture to chill and set for about 30 minutes.
5. Once the mixture is firm and set, remove it from the refrigerator, and using a sharp knife, cut it into bars.
6. Store any leftover bars in the refrigerator in an airtight container.

Nutritional Facts:
Calories 190 | Carbohydrates 3.9 g | Protein 5.1 g | Fat 18 g | Sodium 105 mg

Chapter 8: Drinks and Smoothies Recipes

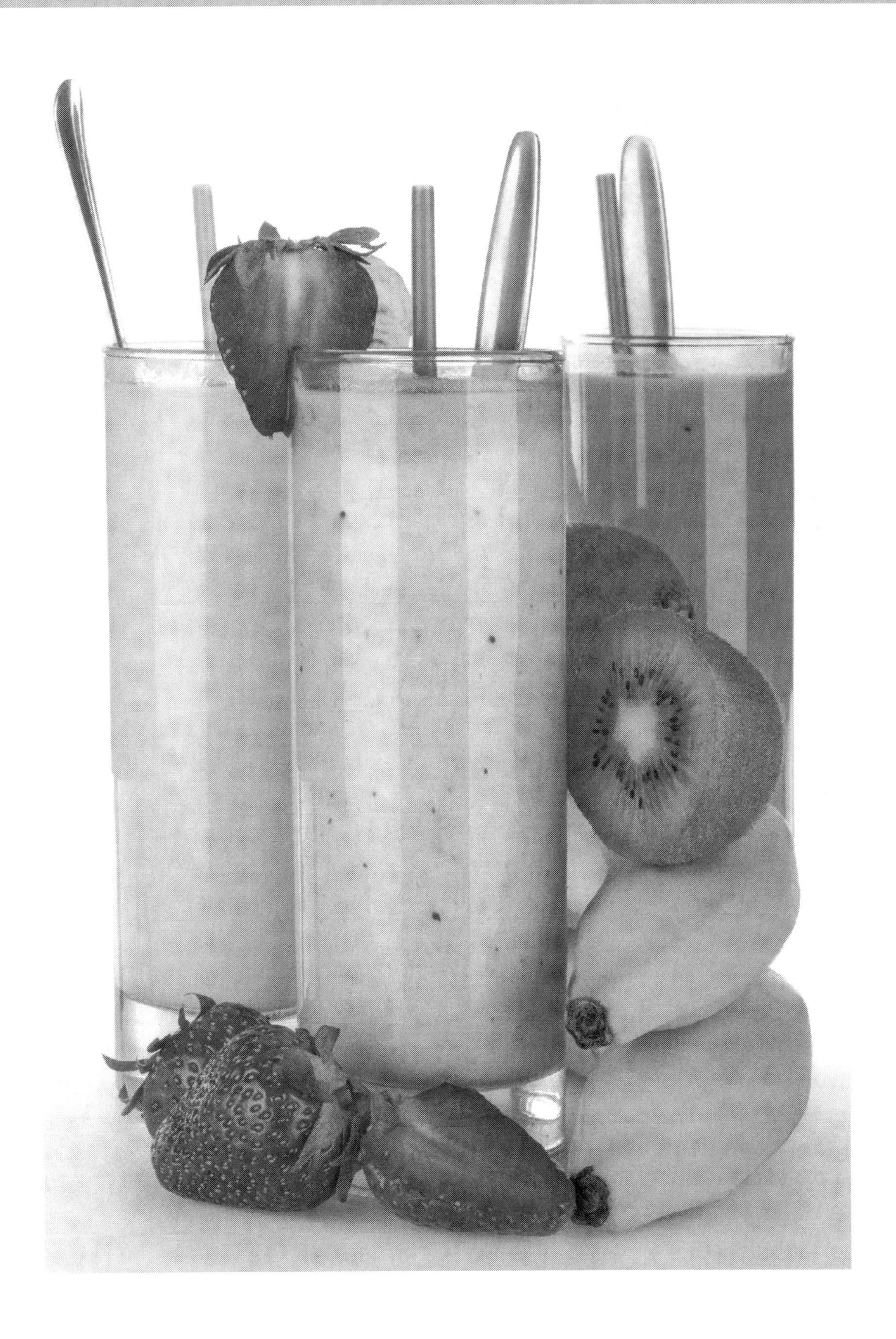

8.1. Strawberry and Chocolate Shake

Ready in:

- ➢ Prep: 10 minutes
- ➢ Cook: 0 minutes
- ➢ Serving: 1

What you need:

- semi-skimmed milk (100 mL)
- 25 g live Greek yogurt (full fat)
- 100g strawberries (fresh or frozen)
- giant porridge oats (15g)
- 1 date with a soft pit
- a teaspoon of cocoa powder
- tablespoon water (cool)

Instructions

1 In a food grinder, add all Ingredients and mix until smooth. If required, add additional water to get a smooth texture.

Nutritional Facts

Calories 119| Carbohydrates 16 g| Protein 4 g| Fat 1 g| Sodium 10 mg |

8.2. Banana Nutty Shake

Ready In:

- ➢ Prep: 6 Min.
- ➢ Serving Single Portion

What you need:

- 20g live Greek yogurt (full fat)
- semi-skimmed milk (100 mL)
- 1/2 medium bananas, peeled and coarsely chopped (about 50g peeled weight)
- 15g nut butter without sugar made from cashews or almonds
- tablespoons water (cool)

Instructions

1 In a food grinder, add all Ingredients and mix until smooth. If required, add additional water to get a smooth texture.

Nutritional Facts

Calories 214| Carbohydrates 22 g| Protein 1 g| Fat 4 g| Sodium 39 mg |

8.3. Minted Cucumber and Avocado Shake

Ready In:

- ➢ Prep: 15 Min.
- ➢ Cook: Not Provided
- ➢ Yields: 1 Single Portion

What you need:

- 1/2 medium avocados, chopped, skinned, and cut into quarters (about 75 grams)
- 200 g thickly sliced cucumber
- 25 g leaves of young spinach
- 15g full-fat live Greek yogurt
- Fresh mint leaves (12grams)
- 100 ml ice water

Instructions

1 In a food grinder, add all Ingredients and mix until smooth. If required, add additional water to get a smooth texture.

Nutritional Facts

Calories 180| Carbohydrates 26 g| Protein 2 g| Fat 2.2 g| Sodium 11 mg |

8.4. Cashew, Carrot and Orange Shake

Ready In:

- Prep: 20 Min.
- Cook: Not Provided
- Yields: 1 Single Portion

What you need:

- 1/2 medium-size orange, skinned and cut into rough pieces
- 1/2 medium carrots (about 170g), trimmed and thinly sliced
- 15 g cashew nut butter or hazelnut butter with no added sugar
- 125 milliliters of cold water

Instructions

1 In a food grinder, add all Ingredients and mix until smooth. If required, add additional water to get a smooth texture.

Nutritional Facts

Calories 215| Carbohydrates 20 g| Protein 5 g| Fat 1.8 g| Sodium 24 mg |

8.5. Ginger Shake

Ready in:

- Prep: 20 minutes
- Cook: not provided
- Serving: 1

What you need:

- 1 quartered green apple
- 1/2 medium courgette, chopped and finely chopped (about 65g)
- 8g peeled and finely chopped fresh root ginger
- 1/2 tsp turmeric powder
- grams of mixed seeds (sunflower, pumpkin and flax)
- teaspoons extra-virgin olive oil
- 100 mL ice water

Instructions

1 In a food mixing grinder, add all Ingredients and mix until smooth. If required, add additional water to get a smooth texture.

Nutritional Facts

Calories 218| Carbohydrates 36 g| Protein 4 g| Fat 2 g| Sodium 8 mg |

8.6. Gazpacho Shake

Ready in:

- Prep: 15 minutes
- Cook: not provided
- Serving: 1

What you need:

- cucumber, 100g, coarsely chopped
- to 3 healthy vine tomatoes, cut into quarters (about 125g)
- 1/2 red pepper, without seed and chopped
- 1/2 red pepper, without seed and chopped
- 25 g Greek yogurt (full fat)
- g almond flour
- 1 tablespoon pureed tomatoes
- 1 teaspoon extra-virgin olive oil
- tablespoons water (cool)
- to taste with salt and black pepper

Instructions

1 In a food mixing grinder, add all Ingredients and mix until smooth. If required, add additional water to get a smooth texture.

Nutritional Facts

Calories 210| Carbohydrates 20.2 g| Protein 12.8 g| Fat 4.3 g| Sodium 12 mg |

8.7. Chai Smoothie

Ready in:

- Prep: 40 min.
- Cook: not provided
- Serving: 1

What you need:

- ½ cup boiling water
- chai tea bags
- ¼ cup sugar
- cups ice
- ½ cup 1% milk

Instructions

1 Combine boiling water, sugar, and chai tea bags in a small bowl Cover and let the tea infuse for five minutes.
2 Discard tea bags, then refrigerate tea for 30 minutes or thoroughly chill. Place tea, ice, and milk in a blender and process until smooth.
3 Serve immediately.

Nutritional Facts

Calories 210| Carbohydrates 26 g| Protein 3 g| Fat 3 g| Sodium 166 mg |

8.8. Apple Chai Smoothie

Ready in:

- Prep: 5 minutes+ 30 minutes to Steep
- Cook: 5 min.
- Yields: 2

What you need:

- 1 cup rice milk, unsweetened
- 1 teabag
- 1 peeled, shelled, and shredded apple
- quarts of ice

Instructions

1 Cook the rice milk in a moderate saucepan or pot over low heat for at least 5 minutes or until bubbling.
2 Start taking the milk off the heat and infusing the teabag in it. Allow 30 minutes for the milk to settle in the refrigerator with the tea bag, remove the teabag and squeeze delicately to release all flavors.
3 Pour the milk, apple, and ice into a blending machine and mix until smooth.
4 Put the smoothie into two glasses and serve.

Nutritional Facts

Calories 88| Carbohydrates 19 g| Protein 1 g| Fat 4 g| Sodium 55 mg |

8.9. Blueberry-Pineapple Smoothie

Ready in:

- Preparation time: 15 minutes
- Cook time: 0 minutes.
- Servings: 2

What you need:

- 1 cup of blueberries, frozen
- 1/2 cup of Pineapple Clumps
- 1/2 cup of cucumber
- 1/2 apple
- 1/2 cup of water

Instructions

1 Take the blueberries, pineapple, cucumber, apple, and water and whirl till they are vicious and silky in a processor.
2 Spoon the smoothie into two glasses and serve.

Nutritional Facts

Calories 87| Carbohydrates 22 g| Protein 1 g| Fat 1 g| Sodium 60 mg |

8.10. Sunny Pineapple Smoothie

Ready in:

- Prep: 5 min.-Cook: 5 min.
- Servings: 2

What you need:

- 1/2 cup of fresh or frozen pineapple chunks
- 2/3 cup of almond milk
- 1/2 teaspoon of ginger powder
- 1 tablespoon agave syrup

Instructions

1 Assemble a smoothie and spin everything for roughly thirty seconds until and unless it's creamy and silky.
2 Fill a glassful or Mason container midway with the mixture.
3 Serve and have fun.

Nutritional Facts

Calories 114| Carbohydrates 37 g| Protein 1.6 g| Fat 0.36 g| Sodium 3 mg |

8.11. Power Boosting Smoothie

Ready in:

- Prep: 5 min.-Cook: 0 min.
- Servings: 2

What you need:

- ½ cup of water
- ½ cup of non-dairy topping
- scoops of protein powder
- 1½ cups of blueberries

Instructions

1 Assemble a smoothie and spin everything for roughly thirty seconds until and unless it's creamy and silky.
2 Fill a glassful or Mason container midway with the mixture.
3 Serve and have fun.

Nutritional Facts

Calories 242| Carbohydrates 34.2 g| Protein 32.3 g| Fat 7.3 g| Sodium 8 mg |

8.12. Strengthening Smoothie Bowl

Ready in:

- Prep: 5 min.-Cook: 0 min.
- Servings: 2

What you need:

- ¼ cup of blueberries
- ¼ cup of plain yogurt
- 1/3 cup of almond milk
- tablespoons of whey protein (powdered form)
- cups of blueberries

Instructions

1 Insert blueberries into a stand mixer and whizz for roughly 1 minute.
2 Process almond milk, yogurt, and protein powder until the desired consistency is achieved.
3 Divide the mixture evenly between the two bowls. End up serving with fresh blueberries as a garnish.

Nutritional Facts

Calories 176| Carbohydrates 27 g| Protein 15 g| Fat 1.6 g| Sodium 9 mg |

8.13. Pineapple Juice

Ready in:

- Prep: 5 min.-Cook: 0 min.
- Servings: 2

What you need:

- ½ cup of sliced pineapple
- 1 cup of fresh
- cubes of ice

Instructions

1 Whisk all Ingredients in an electric mixer and end up serving over ice.

Nutritional Facts

Calories 135| Carbohydrates 0 g| Protein 0 g| Fat 0 g| Sodium 23 mg |

8.14. Grapefruit Sorbet

Ready in:

- Prep: 10 min.-Cook time: 0 min.
- Servings: 2

What you need:

- ½ cup of granulated sugar
- ¼ cup of water
- 1 fresh thyme sprig

For the sorbet

- Juice of 6 grapefruit
- ¼ cup of thyme syrup

Instructions

1 To make the simple thyme syrup
2 Combine the sugar, water, and thyme in a small frying pan or skillet. Bring to a boil, turn off the heat, and refrigerate the thyme sprig until cold. Strain the thyme sprig from the syrup.
3 To make the sorbet
4 Merge the grapefruit juice and 1/4 cup of simple syrup in a juicer and whisk until creamy. Freeze for 3 to 4 hours, just until firm, in an airtight container. Serve.

Nutritional Facts

Calories 117| Carbohydrates 18.2 g| Protein 22.7 g| Fat 2.6 g| Sodium 12 mg |

8.15. Strawberry Cheesecake Smoothie

Ready in:

- Prep: 5 min.-Cook: 0 min.
- Servings: 2

What you need:

- 1 cup of rice milk
- 1 cup of strawberries
- tablespoons of cream cheese
- ½ teaspoon of honey
- 1 teaspoon of vanilla extract
- ice cubes

Instructions

1 Add all the Ingredients to the blending machine, including rice milk, strawberries, cream cheese, honey, vanilla, and ice cubes, and process until the texture gets smooth.
2 End up serving after processing until soft.

Nutritional Facts

Calories 114| Carbohydrates 13 g| Protein 1 g| Fat 3 g| Sodium 19 mg |

FULL MEALS IN JUST 20 MINUTES

Exclusive Digital Cookbook: A Gift for You!

In an ever-evolving and **increasingly fast-paced world**, finding the time to cook **healthy dishes** can be a challenge. With this in mind, I've crafted a **digital cookbook** for those wishing to follow an **anti-inflammatory diet** but are short on kitchen time.

This cookbook boasts a collection of recipes shaped by three key factors: **adherence** to the anti-inflammatory diet, **speedy preparation**, and **flavor.** Each recipe is crafted to replace a **complete meal,** offering a swift and nourishing solution for those in a hurry.

But that's not all! Beyond the **exclusive recipes** of the digital cookbook, I've also curated for you a selection of recipes from this cookbook that meet these specific requirements. These recipes are perfect for those seeking **practical solutions** without compromising on **nutritional quality.**

Scan the **QR code** or visit the provided **link** to discover these recipes. I hope they serve you well on your journey towards a **balanced diet**. Enjoy your meal!

Direct Link:

https://bit.ly/3ro2Dma

QR CODE:

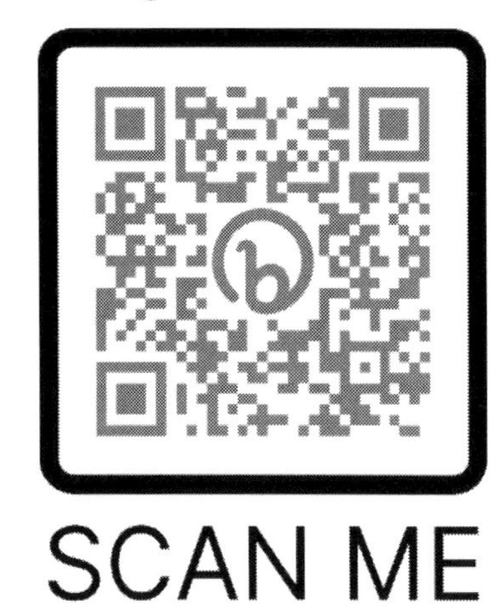

Here's a list of quick recipes, ideal as full meal replacements, found in this cookbook, in addition to those contained in the digital book.

2.3 Blueberry Vanilla Quinoa Porridge

Preparation Time: 1 min-Cook Time: 15 min

Meal Replacement: Breakfast, Snack, Lunch, Dinner

Quinoa is a good protein source, while blueberries provide antioxidants. This recipe can also be adapted for lunch or dinner by adding fresh or dried fruit to boost the protein content.

Nutritional Indicators: High in Protein, Vitamin-Rich, Antioxidant

2.10 Creamy Strawberry Quinoa Delight

Cook Time: 15-20 min.

Meal Replacement: Breakfast, Snack, Lunch, Dinner

Quinoa cooked with coconut milk, natural sweetener, and strawberries. Suitable for various meals.

Nutritional Indicators: Healthy

2.16. Maple-Cinnamon Quinoa Delight

Cook Time: 15 min.

Meal Replacement: Breakfast, Snack, Lunch, Dinner

Quinoa cooked with non-dairy milk, cinnamon, crunchy nuts, and maple or agave syrup. Suitable for various meals.

Nutritional Indicators: Healthy

2.17. Anti-Inflammatory Quinoa Fruit Bowl

Preparation Time: 5 min.-Assembly Time: 5 min.

Meal Replacement: Breakfast, Snack, Lunch, Dinner

A bowl of quinoa cooked with almond milk, bananas, cherries, blueberries, chopped nuts, and turmeric maple syrup for an anti-inflammatory touch. Suitable for various meals.

Nutritional Indicators: Healthy

3.1. Crunchy Chicken Salad

Cooking Time: None, just chilling

Meal Replacement: Lunch, Dinner

This crunchy chicken salad provides a source of lean protein from chicken and boiled eggs, while veggies like onion and celery add vitamins and fiber. It's a light and healthy option for lunch or dinner.

Nutritional Indicators: Healthy

3.2. Anti-Inflammatory Blackened Chicken with Quail

Cooking Time: 20 min.

Meal Replacement: Lunch, Dinner

This dish delivers an explosion of anti-inflammatory flavors thanks to spices like turmeric, ginger, and white pepper. Lean proteins from chicken and quail support protein needs. Great for lunch or dinner.

Nutritional Indicators: Healthy

3.3. Spicy Paprika Lamb Chops

Cooking Time: 10 min.

Meal Replacement: Lunch, Dinner

These lamb chops are loaded with flavor from a mix of spicy seasonings, including paprika and chili. Lamb protein supports muscle building and satiety. Perfect for lunch or dinner.

Nutritional Indicators: Healthy (S)

3.4. Almond Chicken

Cooking Time: 15 min.

Meal Replacement: Lunch, Dinner

Benefits: This dish offers a crispy, flavorful take on chicken due to its almond flour coating. Almonds bring in healthy fats while chicken provides protein for muscle maintenance. Great for lunch or dinner.

Nutritional Indicators: Healthy

3.6. Toasted Sesame Grilled Chicken

Preparation Time: 10 min.-Grilling Time: 8 min.

Meal Replacement: Lunch, Dinner

This grilled chicken with toasted sesame seeds offers a combination of intense flavors from sesame, ginger, and soy sauce. Chicken provides lean protein, and the flavorful ingredients make it a delicious option for lunch or dinner.

Nutritional Indicators: High Protein, Anti-inflammatory, Vitamin-Rich

3.7. Dreamy Lemon-Tarragon Chicken

Cooking Time: 15 min.

Meal Replacement: Lunch, Dinner

This lemon and tarragon chicken dish delivers a fresh, aromatic flavor. Chicken and mushrooms provide protein and nutrients, while coconut cream gives a creamy texture. Perfect for lunch or dinner.

Nutritional Indicators: Anti-inflammatory, Vitamin-Rich

3.11. Tender Chicken in Sweet and Sour Sauce

Cooking Time: 7 min.

Meal Replacement: Dinner

This sweet and sour chicken offers a blend of sweetness and tanginess. Chicken provides protein, while the addition of fruit and vegetables like bell peppers and pineapple adds nutrients and flavor. Perfect for a quick dinner.

Nutritional Indicators: High Protein, Anti-inflammatory, Vitamin-Rich

3.16. Chicken and Veggie Soba Noodles

Cooking Time: 10 min.

Meal Replacement: Lunch, Dinner

This soba noodle dish with chicken and vegetables provides a combination of carbohydrates, protein, and fiber. The chicken and veggies supply essential nutrients. Perfect for a balanced meal.

Nutritional Indicators: Healthy

3.18. Hearty Chicken Stir-Fry

Cooking Time: 20 min.

Meal Replacement: Dinner

This chicken stir-fry offers a combination of lean protein from the chicken and a variety of vegetables. The dish is flavorful and balanced, enhanced by the sauce. Perfect for a nutritious dinner.

Nutritional Indicators: High Protein, Healthy

3.19. Delightful Turkey Flatbread Pizza

Cooking Time: 16 min.

Meal Replacement: Dinner

This turkey pizza provides a lighter, tasty variation compared to traditional pizzas. The turkey provides lean protein, and the veggies add nutrients. Perfect for a delightful dinner.

Nutritional Indicators: Healthy

5.4. Saucy Garlic Greens

Cooking Time: 20 min.

Meal Replacement: Dinner

These greens seasoned with garlic sauce and cashews offer a variety of flavors and textures. The cashews provide healthy fats.

Nutritional Indicators: Healthy

5.5. Pasta with Creamy Broccoli Sauce

Preparation Time: 15-20 min

Cooking Time: Varies

Meal Replacement: Lunch or Dinner

This pasta with creamy broccoli sauce offers a mix of carbs, proteins, and veggies. It's a balanced and flavorful choice.

Nutritional Indicators: Healthy

5.8. Garden Salad

Preparation Time: 10 min.

Meal Replacement: Lunch or Dinner

Benefits: This fresh salad offers a variety of vegetables and proteins from peanut chunks.

Nutritional Indicators: Healthy

5.11. Peas Soup

Cooking Time: 10 min.

Meal Replacement: Lunch

Benefits: This pea soup is rich in plant proteins and has a fresh, light flavor.

Nutritional Indicators: Healthy

5.13. Cauliflower Rice and Coconut

Cooking Time: 15-20 min.

Meal Replacement: Dinner

This coconut cauliflower rice dish is flavorful and light with a spicy kick from sriracha.

Nutritional Indicators: Healthy

5.14. Kale and Garlic Platter

Cooking Time: 12 min.

Meal Replacement: Dinner

This garlic kale dish offers a variety of flavors and can be a great side for a light dinner.

Nutritional Indicators: Healthy

5.15. Blistered Beans and Almond

Cooking Time: 20 min.

Meal Replacement: Dinner

These blistered green beans with almonds provide a contrast of textures and flavors, enriched by the crunchiness of the almonds.

Nutritional Indicators: Healthy

5.16. Cucumber Soup

Preparation Time: 10 min.

Meal Replacement: Lunch

This cucumber soup is light and refreshing, perfect as a cold dish on a hot day.

Nutritional Indicators: Healthy

5.17. Eggplant Salad

Cooking Time: 20 min.

Meal Replacement: Dinner

This eggplant salad offers a mix of flavors and can be a delicious and healthy side.

Nutritional Indicators: Healthy

5.19. Broccoli Blossom

Cooking Time: 10 min.

Meal Replacement: Dinner

This broccoli and red cabbage dish provides a mix of flavors and can be a healthy addition to a light dinner.

Nutritional Indicators: Moderate (due to the use of Parmesan cheese)

5.20. Hot German Cabbage

Cooking Time: 15 min.

Meal Replacement: Dinner

This German-style cabbage dish offers a mix of sweet and sour flavors, perfect for a side dish.

Nutritional Indicators: Moderate (due to the use of honey)

6.1. Juicy Salmon Dish

Cooking Time: 15 min.

Meal Replacement: Lunch, Dinner

A dish rich in proteins and healthy fats, enhanced with vitamins from herbs. Ideal for lunch or dinner.

Nutritional Indicators: Healthy

6.3. Herb Topped Fish

Cooking Time: 20 min.

Meal Replacement: Lunch, Dinner

Rich in protein, healthy fats, and garnished with aromatic herbs for flavor and antioxidants.

Nutritional Indicators: Healthy

6.4. Fish Cakes

Cooking Time: 15 min.

Meal Replacement: Lunch, Dinner

Benefits: Protein from the fish and carbs from potatoes, combined into tasty patties. Ideal for lunch or dinner.

Nutritional Indicators: Healthy, : High Protein

6.5. Salmon Pasta with Butter

Cooking Time: 15 min.

Meal Replacement: Lunch

Protein from salmon and carbs from pasta, enriched with butter. Great for lunch.

Nutritional Indicators: Moderate, High Protein

6.6. Salmon with Pineapple Salsa

Cooking Time: 20 min.

Meal Replacement: Lunch, Dinner

Protein from salmon and vitamins from the pineapple salsa. Excellent for lunch or dinner.

Nutritional Indicators: Healthy, High Protein

Tip: Pair with a serving of leafy greens to add fiber and nutrients.

6.7. Smoked Haddock with Lentils

Cooking Time: 20 min.

Meal Replacement: Lunch, Dinner

Protein from the fish and fiber from the lentils. A balanced meal.

Nutritional Indicators: Healthy, High Protein

Tip: Serve with a portion of root or leafy vegetables for a complete dish.

6.8. Pan-Fried Fish with Lemon and Parsley

Cooking Time: 20 min.

Meal Replacement: Lunch, Dinner

Protein from the fish and vitamin C from the lemon. Simple and tasty.

Nutritional Indicators: Healthy, High Protein

Tip: Add a colorful salad for a variety of nutrients.

6.9. Crunchy Fish Bites

Cooking Time: 20 min.

Meal Replacement: Lunch, Dinner

Protein from the fish and crunchiness from the nut coating. Perfect for lunch or dinner.

Nutritional Indicators: Healthy, High Protein

Tip: Pair with a serving of steamed or roasted vegetables.

6.13. Turmeric-Infused Shellfish in Wine

Cooking Time: 20 min.

Meal Replacement: Lunch, Dinner

Protein from fish and aromatic flavor from ginger and turmeric. Pairs well with white wine.

Nutritional Indicators: Moderate, High Protein

Suggestion: Pair with a serving of brown rice or quinoa to increase carbohydrate intake.

6.14. Pistachio Fish

Cooking Time: 10 min.

Meal Replacement: Lunch, Dinner

Protein from fish and healthy fats from pistachios. Crispy crust for a tasty dish.

Nutritional Indicators: Healthy, High Protein

Suggestion: Serve with a portion of leafy green vegetables for a complete meal.

6.15. Herb-Crusted Tilapia

Cooking Time: 15 min.

Meal Replacement: Lunch, Dinner

Protein from fish and aromatic flavor from herbs. Crispy crust with a fresh taste.

Nutritional Indicators: Healthy, High Protein

Suggestion: Serve with a serving of quinoa or roasted sweet potatoes.

6.16. Grilled Mahi with Mango Salsa

Cooking Time: 10 min.

Meal Replacement: Lunch, Dinner

Protein from fish and freshness from the mango salsa. A light and vibrant dish.

Nutritional Indicators: Healthy, High Protein

Suggestion: Pair with a mixed salad for a balanced meal.

6.17. Cod in Ginger and Turmeric Broth

Cooking Time: 20 min.

Meal Replacement: Lunch, Dinner

Protein from fish and anti-inflammatory properties from ginger and turmeric. Aromatic and flavorful broth.

Nutritional Indicators: Moderate, High Protein

Suggestion: Serve with a serving of steamed vegetables or a small portion of brown rice.

8.3. Minted Cucumber and Avocado Shake

Preparation Time: 15 min.

Meal Replacement: Lunch, Dinner

Avocado provides healthy fats, while cucumber adds hydration. Spinach leaves and mint offer additional nutrients. Perfect for a balanced meal.

Nutritional Indicators: Healthy

8.4. Cashew, Carrot and Orange Shake

Preparation Time: 20 min.

Meal Replacement: Lunch, Dinner

This shake combines protein from nut butters with fiber from carrots and vitamin C from orange. It's a nutritious choice for a complete meal.

Nutritional Indicators: Moderate

8.5. Ginger Shake

Preparation Time: 20 min.

Meal Replacement: Breakfast, Lunch

Ginger offers anti-inflammatory properties, while apple and zucchini add nutrients. Perfect to start the day or as a light meal.

Nutritional Indicators: Healthy

8.6. Gazpacho Shake

Preparation Time: 15 min.

Meal Replacement: Lunch, Dinner

This vegetable-rich shake offers antioxidants and vitamins. Ideal for a healthy lunch break or a light dinner.

Nutritional Indicators: Healthy

GET YOUR BONUSES

Dear Valued Reader,

First and foremost, **thank you** for choosing and investing in this book. Your trust and commitment to a healthier lifestyle means the world to me.

You may have noticed that the book, although filled with delightful recipes, has limited images.

This was a deliberate choice. While I understand that vibrant, colorful images can enhance the reading experience, printing them in black and white wouldn't truly capture the essence and vibrancy of the dishes. Moreover, including color images would have made the book considerably more expensive.

I genuinely hope you understand this decision was made with the best intentions in mind: to provide you with valuable content at an affordable price.

To show my appreciation and to further aid you on your journey to wellness, I've crafted a special bonus exclusively for you:

"Flame-Off: Your 5-Step No-Stress Anti-Inflammatory Blueprint"

Click on the link provided, or scan the QR code, to download your exclusive guide inside it you will also find a very useful **Shopping Card.** This is my heartfelt way of saying **thank you**.

Your trust and understanding are deeply cherished. Here's to a healthier, brighter you!

Warmly, [*Alison Tenny*]

SCAN THE QR CODE OR COPY THE LINK http://bit.ly/46KrEqP

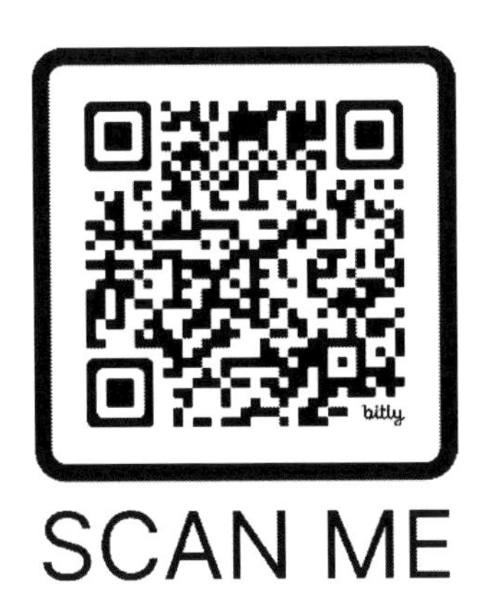

SCAN ME

Meal Plan

WEEK 1

MONDAY:

- **Breakfast:** Blueberry Vanilla Quinoa Porridge (2.3)
- **Lunch:** Crunchy Chicken Salad (3.1)
- **Snack:** Healthy Golden Eggplant Fries (5.1)
- **Dinner:** Juicy Salmon Dish (6.1)

TUESDAY:

- **Breakfast:** Banana Pancake Muffins (2.6)

1. **Lunch:** Cream of Mushroom Soup (4.13)
2. **Snack:** Strawberry-Mango Parfaits with Ginger Topping (7.3)

- **Dinner:** Herb-Crusted Tilapia (6.15)

WEDNESDAY:

- **Breakfast:** Rise & Shine Rice Porridge (2.15)
- **Lunch:** Spicy Cabbage Dish (5.10)
- **Snack:** Cocoa Fat Bombs (7.15)
- **Dinner:** Mediterranean Fish Bake (6.10)

THURSDAY:

- **Breakfast:** Maple-Cinnamon Quinoa Delight (2.16)
- **Lunch:** Zesty Blackberry Chicken Wings (3.5)
- **Snack:** Blackberry Cobbler (7.7)
- **Dinner:** Cream of Watercress Soup (4.10)

FRIDAY:

- **Breakfast:** Cinnamon-Flax Morning Bread (2.7)
- **Lunch:** Creamy Thyme Carrot Soup (4.4)
- **Snack:** Almond Peanut Butter Bars (7.16)
- **Dinner:** Ginger and Chili Baked Fish (6.11)

SATURDAY:

- **Breakfast**: Sunny Morning Coconut Pancakes (2.14)
- **Lunch:** Pesto Pasta with Cream (5.7)
- **Snack:** Strawberry Cheesecake Smoothie (8.14)
- **Dinner:** Fish with Peppers (6.2)

SUNDAY:

- **Breakfast:** Creamy Strawberry Quinoa Delight (2.10)
- **Lunch:** Mesmerizing Lentil Soup (4.12)
- **Snack**: Antojitos (7.14)
- **Dinner:** Smoked Haddock with Lentils (6.7)

WEEK 2

MONDAY:

- **Breakfast:** Buckwheat Ginger Granola (2.4)
- **Lunch**: Basil Zucchini Spaghetti (5.12)
- **Snack:** Lemon Ricotta Pie (7.9)
- **Dinner:** Turmeric-Infused Shellfish in Wine (6.13)

TUESDAY:

- **Breakfast:** Veggie Morning Delight (2.8)
- **Lunch:** Eggplant Vegetable Soup (4.1)
- **Snack:** Almond Peanut Butter Bars (7.16)
- **Dinner:** Toasted Sesame Grilled Chicken (3.6)

WEDNESDAY:

- **Breakfast:** Creamy Asparagus Soup (4.15)
- **Lunch:** Egg Kale with Casserole (2.1)
- **Snack:** Blueberries and Cream Ice Pops (7.1)
- **Dinner:** Herb Topped Fish (6.3)

THURSDAY:

- **Breakfast:** Strawberry and Chocolate Shake (8.1)
- **Lunch:** Ground Beef and Rice Soup (4.19)
- **Snack:** Strawberry Cheesecake Smoothie (8.14)
- **Dinner:** Spicy Paprika Lamb Chops (3.3)

FRIDAY:

- **Breakfast:** Minted Cucumber and Avocado Shake (8.3)
- **Lunch:** Roasted Vegetable Soup (4.14)
- **Snack:** Healthy Protein Bars (7.17)
- **Dinner:** Grilled Mahi Mahi with Mango Salsa (6.16)

SATURDAY:

- **Breakfast:** Banana Nutty Shake (8.2)
- **Lunch:** Cream of Corn Soup (4.5)
- **Snack:** Gazpacho Shake (8.6)
- **Dinner:** Cod in Ginger and Turmeric Broth (6.17)

SUNDAY:

- **Breakfast:** Zucchini Pancakes (2.6)
- **Lunch:** Rice and Chicken Soup (4.7)
- **Snack:** Strawberry-Mango Parfaits with Ginger Topping (7.3)
- **Dinner:** Chicken Fingers with a Honeyed Dip (3.13)

WEEK 3

MONDAY:

- **Breakfast:** Pesto Pasta with Cream (5.7)
- **Lunch:** Cream of Mushroom Soup (4.13)
- **Snack:** Cocoa Fat Bombs (7.15)
- **Dinner:** Juicy Salmon Dish (6.1)

TUESDAY:

- **Breakfast:** Spicy Cabbage Dish (5.10)
- **Lunch:** Turkey Bulgur Soup (4.18)
- **Snack:** Blackberry Cobbler (7.7)
- **Dinner:** Golden Oven-Crisped Chicken (3.10)

WEDNESDAY:

- **Breakfast:** Blueberry-Pineapple Smoothie (8.9)
- **Lunch:** Hearty Homestyle Meat Loaf (3.8)
- **Snack:** Strawberry Cheesecake Smoothie (8.14)
- **Dinner:** Cod in Ginger and Turmeric Broth (6.17)

THURSDAY:

- **Breakfast:** Rustic Root Veggie & Egg Bake (2.9)
- **Lunch:** Delightful Turkey Flatbread Pizza (3.19)
- **Snack:** Almond Peanut Butter Bars (7.16)
- **Dinner:** Toasted Sesame Grilled Chicken (3.6)

FRIDAY:

- **Breakfast:** Sunny Pineapple Smoothie (8.10)
- **Lunch:** Eggplant Vegetable Soup (4.1)
- **Snack:** Strawberry-Mango Parfaits with Ginger Topping (7.3)
- **Dinner:** Smoked Haddock with Lentils (6.7)

SATURDAY:

- **Breakfast:** Creamy Strawberry Quinoa Delight (2.10)
- **Lunch:** Creamy Thyme Carrot Soup (4.4)
- **Snack:** Antojitos (7.14)
- **Dinner:** Grilled Mahi Mahi with Mango Salsa (6.16)

SUNDAY:

- **Breakfast:** Maple-Cinnamon Quinoa Delight (2.16)
- **Lunch:** Ground Beef and Rice Soup (4.19)
- **Snack:** Lemon Ricotta Pie (7.9)
- **Dinner:** Ginger and Chili Baked Fish (6.11)

WEEK 4

MONDAY:

- **Breakfast:** Buckwheat Ginger Granola (2.4)
- **Lunch:** Cream of Watercress Soup (4.10)
- **Snack:** Blueberries and Cream Ice Pops (7.1)
- **Dinner:** Herb Topped Fish (6.3)

TUESDAY:

- **Breakfast:** Rise & Shine Rice Porridge (2.15)
- **Lunch:** Chicken Fingers with a Honeyed Dip (3.13)
- **Snack:** Healthy Protein Bars (7.17)
- **Dinner:** Mediterranean Fish Bake (6.10)

WEDNESDAY:

- **Breakfast:** Veggie Morning Delight (2.8)
- **Lunch:** Basil Zucchini Spaghetti (5.12)
- **Snack:** Strawberry Lime Dessert (7.5)
- **Dinner:** Crusted Whitefish (6.12)

THURSDAY:

- **Breakfast:** Strawberry and Chocolate Shake (8.1)
- **Lunch:** Roasted Red Pepper and Chicken Crostini (7.12)
- **Snack:** Cocoa Fat Bombs (7.15)
- **Dinner:** Zesty Blackberry Chicken Wings (3.5)

FRIDAY:

- **Breakfast:** Minted Cucumber and Avocado Shake (8.3)
- **Lunch:** Egg Kale with Casserole (2.1)
- **Snack:** Gazpacho Shake (8.6)
- **Dinner:** Golden Oven-Crisped Chicken (3.10)

SATURDAY:

- **Breakfast:** Banana Nutty Shake (8.2)
- **Lunch:** Cream of Corn Soup (4.5)
- **Snack:** Strawberry-Mango Parfaits with Ginger Topping (7.3)
- **Dinner:** Crusted Whitefish (6.12)

SUNDAY:

- **Breakfast:** Rise & Shine Rice Porridge (2.15)
- **Lunch:** Rice and Chicken Soup (4.7)
- **Snack:** Almond Peanut Butter Bars (7.16)
- **Dinner:** Spicy Paprika Lamb Chops (3.3)

WEEK 5

MONDAY:

- **Breakfast:** Blueberry Vanilla Quinoa Porridge (2.3)
- **Lunch:** Eggplant Vegetable Soup (4.1)
- **Snack:** Cashew, Carrot and Orange Shake (8.4)
- **Dinner:** Grilled Mahi Mahi with Mango Salsa (6.16)

TUESDAY:

- **Breakfast:** Banana Pancake Muffins (2.6)
- **Lunch:** Turkey Bulgur Soup (4.18)
- **Snack:** Lemon Ricotta Pie (7.9)
- **Dinner:** Almond Chicken (3.4)

WEDNESDAY:

- **Breakfast:** Rise & Shine Rice Porridge (2.15)
- **Lunch:** Basil Zucchini Spaghetti (5.12)
- **Snack:** Strawberry-Mango Parfaits with Ginger Topping (7.3)
- **Dinner:** Cod in Ginger and Turmeric Broth (6.17)

THURSDAY:

- **Breakfast:** Buckwheat Ginger Granola (2.4)
- **Lunch:** Cream of Mushroom Soup (4.13)
- **Snack:** Blackberry Cobbler (7.7)
- **Dinner:** Steak with a Tender Onion Embrace (3.9)

FRIDAY:

- **Breakfast:** Cinnamon-Flax Morning Bread (2.7)
- **Lunch:** Ground Beef and Rice Soup (4.19)
- **Snack:** Strawberry Cheesecake Smoothie (8.14)
- **Dinner:** Toasted Sesame Grilled Chicken (3.6)

SATURDAY:

- **Breakfast:** Minted Cucumber and Avocado Shake (8.3)
- **Lunch:** French Onion Soup (4.10)
- **Snack:** Antojitos (7.14)
- **Dinner:** Smoked Haddock with Lentils (6.7)

SUNDAY:

- **Breakfast:** Creamy Strawberry Quinoa Delight (2.10)
- **Lunch:** Rice and Chicken Soup (4.7)
- **Snack:** Blueberries and Cream Ice Pops (7.1)
- **Dinner:** Chicken Fingers with a Honeyed Dip (3.13)

WEEK 6

MONDAY:

- **Breakfast:** Buckwheat Ginger Granola (2.4)
- **Lunch:** Cream of Watercress Soup (4.10)
- **Snack:** Strawberry Lime Dessert (7.5)
- **Dinner:** Herb Topped Fish (6.3)

TUESDAY:

- **Breakfast:** Veggie Morning Delight (2.8)
- **Lunch:** Chicken Fingers with a Honeyed Dip (3.13)
- **Snack:** Cocoa Fat Bombs (7.15)
- **Dinner:** Mediterranean Fish Bake (6.10)

WEDNESDAY:

- **Breakfast:** Strawberry and Chocolate Shake (8.1)
- **Lunch:** Delightful Turkey Flatbread Pizza (3.19)
- **Snack:** Strawberry-Mango Parfaits with Ginger Topping (7.3)
- **Dinner:** Crusted Whitefish (6.12)

THURSDAY:

- **Breakfast:** Rustic Root Veggie & Egg Bake (2.9)
- **Lunch:** Egg Kale with Casserole (2.1)
- **Snack:** Gazpacho Shake (8.6)
- **Dinner:** Golden Oven-Crisped Chicken (3.10)

FRIDAY:

- **Breakfast:** Minted Cucumber and Avocado Shake (8.3)
- **Lunch:** Roasted Red Pepper and Chicken Crostini (7.12)
- **Snack:** Strawberry Cheesecake Smoothie (8.14)
- **Dinner:** Zesty Blackberry Chicken Wings (3.5)

SATURDAY:

- **Breakfast:** Banana Nutty Shake (8.2)
- **Lunch:** Cream of Corn Soup (4.5)
- **Snack:** Blueberries and Cream Ice Pops (7.1)
- **Dinner:** Crusted Whitefish (6.12)

SUNDAY:

- **Breakfast:** Zucchini Pancakes (2.6)
- **Lunch:** Rice and Chicken Soup (4.7)
- **Snack:** Almond Peanut Butter Bars (7.16)
- **Dinner:** Spicy Paprika Lamb Chops (3.3)

WEEK 7

MONDAY:

- **Breakfast:** Blueberry Vanilla Quinoa Porridge (2.3)
- **Lunch:** Eggplant Vegetable Soup (4.1)
- **Snack:** Cashew, Carrot and Orange Shake (8.4)
- **Dinner:** Grilled Mahi Mahi with Mango Salsa (6.16)

TUESDAY:

- **Breakfast:** Banana Pancake Muffins (2.6)
- **Lunch:** Turkey Bulgur Soup (4.18)
- **Snack:** Lemon Ricotta Pie (7.9)
- **Dinner:** Almond Chicken (3.4)

WEDNESDAY:

- **Breakfast:** Rise & Shine Rice Porridge (2.15)
- **Lunch:** Basil Zucchini Spaghetti (5.12)
- **Snack:** Strawberry-Mango Parfaits with Ginger Topping (7.3)
- **Dinner:** Cod in Ginger and Turmeric Broth (6.17)

THURSDAY:

- **Breakfast:** Buckwheat Ginger Granola (2.4)
- **Lunch:** Cream of Mushroom Soup (4.13)
- **Snack:** Blackberry Cobbler (7.7)
- **Dinner:** Steak with a Tender Onion Embrace (3.9)

FRIDAY:

- **Breakfast:** Cinnamon-Flax Morning Bread (2.7)
- **Lunch:** Ground Beef and Rice Soup (4.19)
- **Snack:** Strawberry Cheesecake Smoothie (8.14)
- **Dinner:** Toasted Sesame Grilled Chicken (3.6)

SATURDAY:

- **Breakfast:** Minted Cucumber and Avocado Shake (8.3)
- **Lunch:** French Onion Soup (4.10)
- **Snack:** Antojitos (7.14)
- **Dinner:** Smoked Haddock with Lentils (6.7)

SUNDAY:

- **Breakfast:** Creamy Strawberry Quinoa Delight (2.10)
- **Lunch:** Rice and Chicken Soup (4.7)
- **Snack:** Blueberries and Cream Ice Pops (7.1)
- **Dinner:** Chicken Fingers with a Honeyed Dip (3.13)

WEEK 8

MONDAY:

- **Breakfast:** Creamy Strawberry Quinoa Delight (2.10)
- **Lunch:** Egg Kale with Casserole (2.1)
- **Snack:** Blueberries and Cream Ice Pops (7.1)
- **Dinner:** Grilled Mahi Mahi with Mango Salsa (6.16)

TUESDAY:

- **Breakfast:** Banana Pancake Muffins (2.6)
- **Lunch:** Cream of Mushroom Soup (4.13)
- **Snack:** Strawberry-Mango Parfaits with Ginger Topping (7.3)
- **Dinner:** Almond Chicken (3.4)

WEDNESDAY:

- **Breakfast:** Rise & Shine Rice Porridge (2.15)
- **Lunch:** Chicken Fingers with a Honeyed Dip (3.13)
- **Snack:** Cocoa Fat Bombs (7.15)
- **Dinner:** Herb Topped Fish (6.3)

THURSDAY:

- **Breakfast:** Maple-Cinnamon Quinoa Delight (2.16)
- **Lunch:** Delightful Turkey Flatbread Pizza (3.19)
- **Snack:** Strawberry Lime Dessert (7.5)
- **Dinner:** Toasted Sesame Grilled Chicken (3.6)

FRIDAY:

- **Breakfast:** Cinnamon-Flax Morning Bread (2.7)
- **Lunch:** Roasted Red Pepper and Chicken Crostini (7.12)
- **Snack:** Antojitos (7.14)
- **Dinner:** Zesty Blackberry Chicken Wings (3.5)

SATURDAY:

- **Breakfast:** Sunny Pineapple Smoothie (8.10)
- **Lunch:** Cream of Corn Soup (4.5)
- **Snack:** Strawberry Cheesecake Smoothie (8.14)
- **Dinner:** Smoked Haddock with Lentils (6.7)

SUNDAY:

- **Breakfast:**Banana Pancake Muffins (2.6)
- **Lunch:** Rice and Chicken Soup (4.7)
- **Snack:** Almond Peanut Butter Bars (7.16)
- **Dinner:** Spicy Paprika Lamb Chops (3.3)

WEEK 9

MONDAY:

- **Breakfast:** Creamy Strawberry Quinoa Delight (2.10)
- **Lunch:** Eggplant Vegetable Soup (4.1)
- **Snack:** Cashew, Carrot and Orange Shake (8.4)
- **Dinner:** Grilled Mahi Mahi with Mango Salsa (6.16)

TUESDAY:

- **Breakfast:** Banana Pancake Muffins (2.6)
- **Lunch:** Turkey Bulgur Soup (4.18)
- **Snack:** Lemon Ricotta Pie (7.9)
- **Dinner:** Almond Chicken (3.4)

WEDNESDAY:

- **Breakfast:** Rise & Shine Rice Porridge (2.15)
- **Lunch:** Basil Zucchini Spaghetti (5.12)
- **Snack:** Strawberry-Mango Parfaits with Ginger Topping (7.3)
- **Dinner:** Cod in Ginger and Turmeric Broth (6.17)

THURSDAY:

- **Breakfast:** Buckwheat Ginger Granola (2.4)
- **Lunch:** Cream of Mushroom Soup (4.13)
- **Snack:** Blackberry Cobbler (7.7)
- **Dinner:** Steak with a Tender Onion Embrace (3.9)

FRIDAY:

- **Breakfast:** Cinnamon-Flax Morning Bread (2.7)
- **Lunch:** Ground Beef and Rice Soup (4.19)
- **Snack:** Strawberry Cheesecake Smoothie (8.14)
- **Dinner:** Toasted Sesame Grilled Chicken (3.6)

SATURDAY:

- **Breakfast:** Minted Cucumber and Avocado Shake (8.3)
- **Lunch:** French Onion Soup (4.10)
- **Snack:** Almond Peanut Butter Bars (7.16)
- **Dinner:** Spicy Paprika Lamb Chops (3.3)

SUNDAY:

- **Breakfast:** Creamy Strawberry Quinoa Delight (2.10)
- **Lunch:** Rice and Chicken Soup (4.7)
- **Snack:** Healthy Protein Bars (7.17)
- **Dinner:** Cod in Ginger and Turmeric Broth (6.17)

WEEK 10

MONDAY:

- **Breakfast:** Egg Kale with Casserole (2.1)
- **Lunch:** Cream of Mushroom Soup (4.13)
- **Snack:** Blueberries and Cream Ice Pops (7.1)
- **Dinner:** Mediterranean Fish Bake (6.10)

TUESDAY:

- **Breakfast:** Banana Pancake Muffins (2.6)
- **Lunch:** Turkey Bulgur Soup (4.18)
- **Snack:** Lemon Ricotta Pie (7.9)
- **Dinner:** Almond Chicken (3.4)

WEDNESDAY:

- **Breakfast:** Rise & Shine Rice Porridge (2.15)
- **Lunch:** Basil Zucchini Spaghetti (5.12)
- **Snack:** Strawberry-Mango Parfaits with Ginger Topping (7.3)
- **Dinner:** Cod in Ginger and Turmeric Broth (6.17)

THURSDAY:

- **Breakfast:** Buckwheat Ginger Granola (2.4)
- **Lunch:** Cream of Watercress Soup (4.10)
- **Snack:** Blackberry Cobbler (7.7)
- **Dinner:** Steak with a Tender Onion Embrace (3.9)

FRIDAY:

- **Breakfast:** Cinnamon-Flax Morning Bread (2.7)
- **Lunch:** Ground Beef and Rice Soup (4.19)
- **Snack:** Strawberry Cheesecake Smoothie (8.14)
- **Dinner:** Toasted Sesame Grilled Chicken (3.6)

SATURDAY:

- **Breakfast:** Minted Cucumber and Avocado Shake (8.3)
- **Lunch:** French Onion Soup (4.10)
- **Snack:** Almond Peanut Butter Bars (7.16)
- **Dinner:** Herb-Crusted Tilapia (6.15)

SUNDAY:

- **Breakfast:** Creamy Strawberry Quinoa Delight (2.10)
- **Lunch:** Rice and Chicken Soup (4.7)
- **Snack:** Healthy Protein Bars (7.17)
- **Dinner:** Cod in Ginger and Turmeric Broth (6.17)

WEEK 11

MONDAY:

- **Breakfast:** Blueberry Vanilla Quinoa Porridge (2.3)
- **Lunch:** Crunchy Chicken Salad (3.1)
- **Snack:** Strawberry-Mango Parfaits with Ginger Topping (7.3)
- **Dinner:** Juicy Salmon Dish (6.1)

TUESDAY:

- **Breakfast:** Rustic Root Veggie & Egg Bake (2.9)
- **Lunch:** Eggplant Vegetable Soup (4.1)
- **Snack:** Cocoa Fat Bombs (7.15)
- **Dinner:** Herb Topped Fish (6.3)

WEDNESDAY:

- **Breakfast:** Banana Pancake Muffins (2.6)
- **Lunch:** Cream of Mushroom Soup (4.13)
- **Snack:** Antojitos (7.14)
- **Dinner:** Zesty Blackberry Chicken Wings (3.5)

THURSDAY:

- **Breakfast:** Maple-Cinnamon Quinoa Delight (2.16)
- **Lunch:** Cream of Corn Soup (4.5)
- **Snack:** Strawberry Cheesecake Smoothie (8.14)
- **Dinner:** Salmon with Pineapple Salsa (6.6)

FRIDAY:

- **Breakfast:** Triple Berry Steel Cut Oats (2.5)
- **Lunch:** Delightful Turkey Flatbread Pizza (3.19)
- **Snack:** Lemon Ricotta Pie (7.9)
- **Dinner:** Turmeric-Infused Shellfish in Wine (6.13)

SATURDAY:

- **Breakfast:** Minted Cucumber and Avocado Shake (8.3)
- **Lunch:** French Onion Soup (4.10)
- **Snack:** Almond Peanut Butter Bars (7.16)
- **Dinner:** Spicy Paprika Lamb Chops (3.3)

SUNDAY:

- **Breakfast:** Creamy Strawberry Quinoa Delight (2.10)
- **Lunch:** Rice and Chicken Soup (4.7)
- **Snack:** Healthy Protein Bars (7.17)
- **Dinner:** Cod in Ginger and Turmeric Broth (6.17)

WEEK 12

MONDAY:

- **Breakfast:** Cinnamon-Flax Morning Bread (2.7)
- **Lunch:** Egg Kale with Casserole (2.1)
- **Snack:** Blueberries and Cream Ice Pops (7.1)
- **Dinner:** Mediterranean Fish Bake (6.10)

TUESDAY:

- **Breakfast:** Veggie Morning Delight (2.8)
- **Lunch:** Cream of Watercress Soup (4.11)
- **Snack:** Strawberry-Mango Parfaits with Ginger Topping (7.3)
- **Dinner:** Almond Chicken (3.4)

WEDNESDAY:

- **Breakfast:** Rise & Shine Rice Porridge (2.15)
- **Lunch:** Ground Beef and Rice Soup (4.19)
- **Snack:** Cocoa Fat Bombs (7.15)
- **Dinner:** Salmon Pasta with Butter (6.5)

THURSDAY:

- **Breakfast:** Banana Pancake Muffins (2.6)
- **Lunch:** Cream of Corn Soup (4.5)
- **Snack:** Antojitos (7.14)
- **Dinner:** Grilled Mahi Mahi with Mango Salsa (6.16)

FRIDAY:

- **Breakfast:** Strawberry and Chocolate Shake (8.1)
- **Lunch:** Delightful Turkey Flatbread Pizza (3.19)
- **Snack:** Lemon Ricotta Pie (7.9)
- **Dinner:** Zesty Blackberry Chicken Wings (3.5)

SATURDAY:

- **Breakfast:** Minted Cucumber and Avocado Shake (8.3)
- **Lunch:** French Onion Soup (4.10)
- **Snack:** Almond Peanut Butter Bars (7.16)
- **Dinner:** Herb-Crusted Tilapia (6.15)

SUNDAY:

- **Breakfast:** Creamy Strawberry Quinoa Delight (2.10)
- **Lunch:** Rice and Chicken Soup (4.7)
- **Snack:** Healthy Protein Bars (7.17)
- Dinner: Cod in Ginger and Turmeric Broth (6.17)

WEEK 13

MONDAY:

- **Breakfast:** Blueberry Vanilla Quinoa Porridge (2.3)
- **Lunch:** Crunchy Chicken Salad (3.1)
- **Snack:** Strawberry-Mango Parfaits with Ginger Topping (7.3)
- **Dinner:** Juicy Salmon Dish (6.1)

TUESDAY:

- **Breakfast:** Rustic Root Veggie & Egg Bake (2.9)
- **Lunch:** Eggplant Vegetable Soup (4.1)
- **Snack:** Cocoa Fat Bombs (7.15)
- **Dinner:** Herb Topped Fish (6.3)

WEDNESDAY:

- Breakfast: Banana Pancake Muffins (2.6)
- **Lunch:** Cream of Mushroom Soup (4.13)
- **Snack:** Antojitos (7.14)
- **Dinner:** Zesty Blackberry Chicken Wings (3.5)

THURSDAY:

- **Breakfast:** Maple-Cinnamon Quinoa Delight (2.16)
- **Lunch:** Cream of Corn Soup (4.5)
- **Snack:** Strawberry Cheesecake Smoothie (8.14)
- **Dinner:** Salmon with Pineapple Salsa (6.6)

FRIDAY:

- **Breakfast:** Triple Berry Steel Cut Oats (2.5)
- **Lunch:** Delightful Turkey Flatbread Pizza (3.19)
- **Snack:** Lemon Ricotta Pie (7.9)
- **Dinner:** Turmeric-Infused Shellfish in Wine (6.13)

SATURDAY:

- **Breakfast:** Minted Cucumber and Avocado Shake (8.3)
- **Lunch:** French Onion Soup (4.10)
- **Snack:** Almond Peanut Butter Bars (7.16)
- **Dinner:** Spicy Paprika Lamb Chops (3.3)

SUNDAY:

- **Breakfast:** Creamy Strawberry Quinoa Delight (2.10)
- **Lunch:** Rice and Chicken Soup (4.7)
- **Snack:** Healthy Protein Bars (7.17)
- **Dinner:** Cod in Ginger and Turmeric Broth (6.17)

WEEK 14

MONDAY:

- **Breakfast:** Egg Kale with Casserole (2.1)
- **Lunch:** Cream of Mushroom Soup (4.13)
- **Snack:** Blueberries and Cream Ice Pops (7.1)
- **Dinner:** Mediterranean Fish Bake (6.10)

TUESDAY:

- **Breakfast:** Veggie Morning Delight (2.8)
- **Lunch:** Cream of Watercress Soup (4.11)
- **Snack:** Strawberry-Mango Parfaits with Ginger Topping (7.3)
- **Dinner:** Almond Chicken (3.4)

WEDNESDAY:

- **Breakfast:** Rise & Shine Rice Porridge (2.15)
- **Lunch:** Ground Beef and Rice Soup (4.19)
- **Snack:** Cocoa Fat Bombs (7.15)
- **Dinner:** Salmon Pasta with Butter (6.5)

THURSDAY:

- **Breakfast:** Banana Pancake Muffins (2.6)
- **Lunch:** Cream of Corn Soup (4.5)
- **Snack:** Antojitos (7.14)
- **Dinner:** Grilled Mahi Mahi with Mango Salsa (6.16)

FRIDAY:

- **Breakfast:** Strawberry and Chocolate Shake (8.1)
- **Lunch:** Delightful Turkey Flatbread Pizza (3.19)
- **Snack:** Lemon Ricotta Pie (7.9)
- **Dinner:** Zesty Blackberry Chicken Wings (3.5)

SATURDAY:

- **Breakfast:** Minted Cucumber and Avocado Shake (8.3)
- **Lunch:** French Onion Soup (4.10)
- **Snack:** Almond Peanut Butter Bars (7.16)
- **Dinner:** Herb-Crusted Tilapia (6.15)

SUNDAY:

- **Breakfast:** Creamy Strawberry Quinoa Delight (2.10)
- **Lunch:** Rice and Chicken Soup (4.7)
- **Snack:** Healthy Protein Bars (7.17)
- **Dinner:** Cod in Ginger and Turmeric Broth (6.17)

WEEK 15

MONDAY:

- **Breakfast:** Blueberry Vanilla Quinoa Porridge (2.3)
- **Lunch:** Crunchy Chicken Salad (3.1)
- **Snack:** Strawberry-Mango Parfaits with Ginger Topping (7.3)
- **Dinner:** Juicy Salmon Dish (6.1)

TUESDAY:

- **Breakfast:** Rustic Root Veggie & Egg Bake (2.9)
- **Lunch:** Eggplant Vegetable Soup (4.1)
- **Snack:** Cocoa Fat Bombs (7.15)
- **Dinner:** Herb Topped Fish (6.3)

WEDNESDAY:

- **Breakfast:** Banana Pancake Muffins (2.6)
- **Lunch:** Cream of Mushroom Soup (4.13)
- **Snack:** Antojitos (7.14)
- **Dinner:** Zesty Blackberry Chicken Wings (3.5)

THURSDAY:

- **Breakfast:** Maple-Cinnamon Quinoa Delight (2.16)
- **Lunch:** Cream of Corn Soup (4.5)
- **Snack:** Strawberry Cheesecake Smoothie (8.14)
- **Dinner:** Salmon with Pineapple Salsa (6.6)

FRIDAY:

- **Breakfast:** Triple Berry Steel Cut Oats (2.5)
- **Lunch:** Delightful Turkey Flatbread Pizza (3.19)
- **Snack:** Lemon Ricotta Pie (7.9)
- **Dinner:** Turmeric-Infused Shellfish in Wine (6.13)

SATURDAY:

- **Breakfast:** Minted Cucumber and Avocado Shake (8.3)
- **Lunch:** French Onion Soup (4.10)
- **Snack:** Almond Peanut Butter Bars (7.16)
- **Dinner:** Spicy Paprika Lamb Chops (3.3)

SUNDAY:

- **Breakfast:** Creamy Strawberry Quinoa Delight (2.10)
- **Lunch:** Rice and Chicken Soup (4.7)
- **Snack:** Healthy Protein Bars (7.17)
- **Dinner:** Cod in Ginger and Turmeric Broth (6.17)

WEEK 16

MONDAY:

- **Breakfast:** Egg Kale with Casserole (2.1)
- **Lunch:** Cream of Mushroom Soup (4.13)
- **Snack:** Blueberries and Cream Ice Pops (7.1)
- **Dinner:** Mediterranean Fish Bake (6.10)

TUESDAY:

- **Breakfast:** Veggie Morning Delight (2.8)
- **Lunch:** Cream of Watercress Soup (4.11)
- **Snack:** Strawberry-Mango Parfaits with Ginger Topping (7.3)
- **Dinner:** Almond Chicken (3.4)

WEDNESDAY:

- **Breakfast:** Rise & Shine Rice Porridge (2.15)
- **Lunch:** Ground Beef and Rice Soup (4.19)
- **Snack:** Cocoa Fat Bombs (7.15)
- **Dinner:** Salmon Pasta with Butter (6.5)

THURSDAY:

- **Breakfast:** Banana Pancake Muffins (2.6)
- **Lunch:** Cream of Corn Soup (4.5)
- **Snack:** Antojitos (7.14)
- **Dinner:** Grilled Mahi Mahi with Mango Salsa (6.16)

FRIDAY:

- **Breakfast:** Strawberry and Chocolate Shake (8.1)
- **Lunch:** Delightful Turkey Flatbread Pizza (3.19)
- **Snack:** Lemon Ricotta Pie (7.9)
- **Dinner:** Zesty Blackberry Chicken Wings (3.5)

SATURDAY:

- **Breakfast:** Minted Cucumber and Avocado Shake (8.3)
- **Lunch:** French Onion Soup (4.10)
- **Snack:** Almond Peanut Butter Bars (7.16)
- **Dinner:** Herb-Crusted Tilapia (6.15)

SUNDAY:

- **Breakfast:** Creamy Strawberry Quinoa Delight (2.10)
- **Lunch:** Rice and Chicken Soup (4.7)
- **Snack:** Healthy Protein Bars (7.17)
- **Dinner:** Cod in Ginger and Turmeric Broth (6.17)

Measurement Chart

1. Dry Measurement Chart

Teaspoons	Tablespoons	Cups
3	1	1/16
6	2	1/8
12	4	1/4
24	8	1/2
36	12	3/4
48	16	1

Metric	Standard
1 gram	.035 oz
100 grams	3.5 oz
500 grams	17.7 oz
1 kilogram	35 oz

2.Liquid Measurement Chart

Fluid Ounces	Cups	Pints	Quarts	Gallons
8	1	1/2	1/4	1/16
16	2	1	1/2	1/8
32	4	2	1	1/4
64	8	4	2	1/2
128	16	8	4	1

Metric	Standard
1 mL	1/5 tsp
5 mL	1 tsp
15 mL	1 tbsp
240 mL	1 c (8 fl. oz)
1 liter	34 fl. Oz

3. Temperature Conversion

(Degrees) Celsius	(Degrees) Fahrenheit
120	250
160	320
180	350
205	400
220	425

4. Us to Metric Conversion

Standard	Metric
1/5 teaspoon	1 millliter
1 teaspoon	5 millliter
1 tablespoon	15 millliter
1 fl. oz	30 millliter
1 cup	237 millliter
1 pint	473 millliter

Standard	Metric
1 quartz	.95 liter
1 gallon	3.8 liter
1 oz	28 grams
1 pound	454 grams

Made in the USA
Las Vegas, NV
16 November 2023

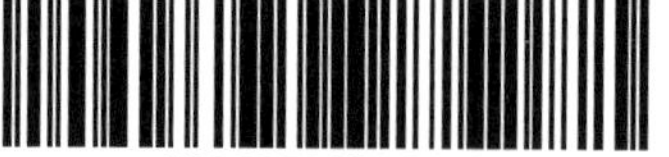
80925764R00059